Holding On for Dear Life

Debbi Huff

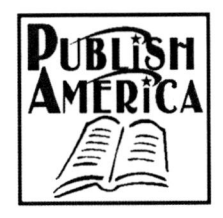

PublishAmerica
Baltimore

© 2007 by Debbi Huff.

All rights reserved. No part of this book may be reproduced, stored in a retrieval system or transmitted in any form or by any means without the prior written permission of the publishers, except by a reviewer who may quote brief passages in a review to be printed in a newspaper, magazine or journal.

First printing

ISBN: 1-4241-5247-X
PUBLISHED BY PUBLISHAMERICA, LLLP
www.publishamerica.com
Baltimore

Printed in the United States of America

Dedication

This book is dedicated to a courageous hero, my son, Chad, and his daughter, Kiersten. It is also dedicated to his brother, Shawn, and his wife and soul mate, Rachael.

May the brave courage, determined fight, enduring strength and faith, joy for life and unconditional love that Chad displayed through his battle never be forgotten and always remain in our minds and hearts forever. He taught us much about life and how to live it. He taught us what is important in life. May we always remember and continue Chad's love for life, nature, kindness, laughter and ability to smile and not complain during hard times.

Born a Hero

He was born to be a hero
At his birth one would never know
Watching ever as he grew
We never even had a clue

He fought small battles of childhood days
As he played in the sunlight's rays
As he grew to be a man
God's course for his life it ran

Pondering upon the past
It did seem he grew too fast
Always with a cup half full
Never letting life be dull

Born from birth to be a hero
Was only God's plan to know
Touching lives upon his way
Bringing joy to every day

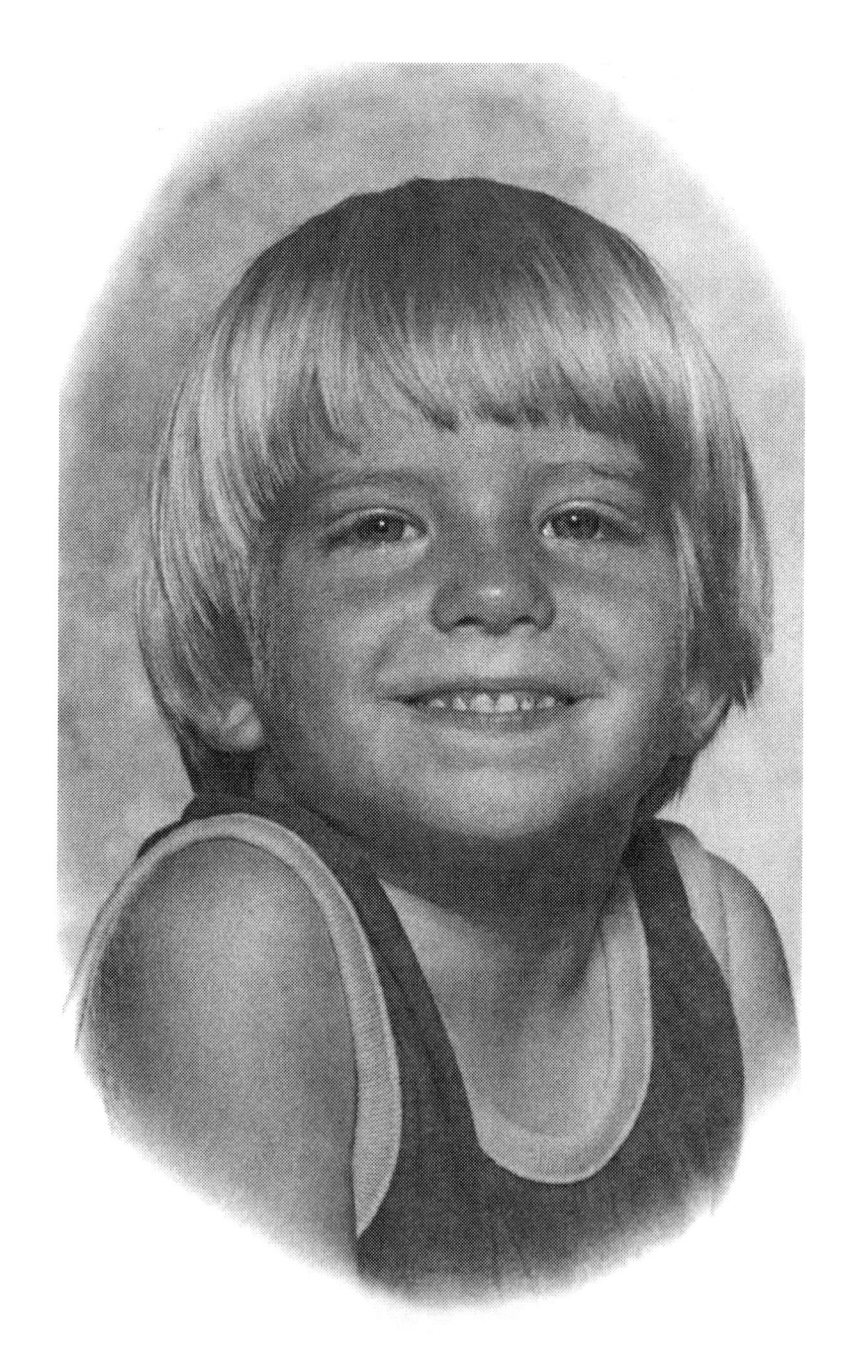

Chad—Our Beloved and Never Forgotten Hero

Foreword

This story is one of courage, faith and strength that are written through a mother's eyes and heart. It is the story of her son's four-year battle with leukemia.

I have been told that "sometimes the truth hurts." I now know that sometimes the truth is almost too painful to bear and may even kill you! The pain that is felt by a cancer patient and their loved ones is more than can be imagined by anyone not wearing those shoes and walking that road.

Acute myelogenous leukemia (AML) is a blood cancer that develops in white blood cells. White blood cells are used by the body to fight infections. The white blood cells do not grow properly when AML develops. This is because of a change or damage to the DNA or genetic matter. Doctors and scientists do not totally understand why the cells are prevented from growing beyond a certain point early in their development. These leukemia cells cannot develop into functional white cells and attack the body instead of helping it. The cells very quickly reproduce in the bone marrow causing minimized production of normal red and white blood cells.

The onset of AML has no specific symptoms. It can be something as simple as a sore throat or sinus problems. It can have a fast onset or slow-developing onset.

Patients with AML get anemic, have a lack of red blood cells that carry oxygen, and become prone to infections due to lack of mature healthy white blood cells to fight off any disease. The patient will bruise and bleed easily due to the lack of platelets along with numerous other symptoms. This can cause the patient to bleed to death. Leukemia cells can also invade other organs in the body, not just the blood.

AML is a common form of leukemia in adults with the average age of patients being sixty-five. More than ten thousand adults are diagnosed with AML in the United States each year. AML affects more men than women and more common in whites than blacks.

Patients with AML usually receive induction chemotherapy drugs as soon as possible after diagnosis. Chemotherapy drugs are used to kill leukemia cells by stopping them from growing to achieve remission (free from leukemia cells) and restore normal blood production. These chemotherapy drugs also kill the normal cells in the body causing the patient to experience side effects including nausea, tiredness and high risk of infection. The patient is then considered neutropenic, meaning their body has no defense from any form of germs.

Most patients' normal blood cell production returns in a few weeks. Remission is determined by microscopic studies of the patient's bone marrow. This is done by doing a bone marrow biopsy. They insert a large needle-shaped device into the patient's hip area that goes down into the bone marrow. Once in remission, further treatments include more chemotherapy or a bone marrow or blood cell transplant.

A bone marrow or blood cell transplant is done by transplanting blood-producing cells into the patient. These cells can be obtained through bone marrow, peripheral blood or umbilical cord blood. The patient must go through pre-transplant chemotherapy and/or radiation to destroy any possible leukemia cells and their immune system. It also destroys healthy cells in the process. The transplant is then done from using the patient's own blood cells or blood cells received from a related or unrelated donor.

A patient receiving blood cells from an outside donor may get graft verses host disease (GVHD). In GVHD the patient's body is attacked by the new immune system in their body that was created by the donor's cells. GVHD can appear soon after transplant or even months or years after transplant. GVHD can be very serious and deadly. Doctors watch transplant patients closely for signs of GVHD so that they can try and control it with medication.

There is a national bone marrow donor program where anyone can get information on how to register to be a bone marrow transplant donor. The registry contains more than five million potential donors or cord blood units to attempt to match the patient's DNA for transplant. The donor and patient must have most of the antigens match for a transplant. More donors are always needed.

I give special thanks and appreciation to the doctors and nursing staff that cared for Chad and helped him in his long battle. They are a special group of people doing a very difficult job. Also to our friends and family that gave us the support and comfort; may your blessings be many.

Chapter 1
June 2001

A Gray Sky

I woke up this morning
And found a gray overcast sky
It came upon me without warning
When you told me you might die

As I hid deep in my room
I could feel the sadness of the gloom
Deep within my soul I knew
The whispers of the chill as the wind blew
My tears fell as mist falls to the ground
But I was too numb to hear a sound

Who put this sadness in my sky
That made my heart feel like it wanted to die
Who took the colorful rainbows and bright sunny day
And left me alone in a dreary haze
Then stepping outside I did discover
The sun was out, it had not died
It is only inside me that it does hide

I woke up this morning
And found a gray overcast sky
A chilly wind came with a warning
And a mist that made the Heavens cry
A haze of fog created a sense of weight
Causing loss of all time and date

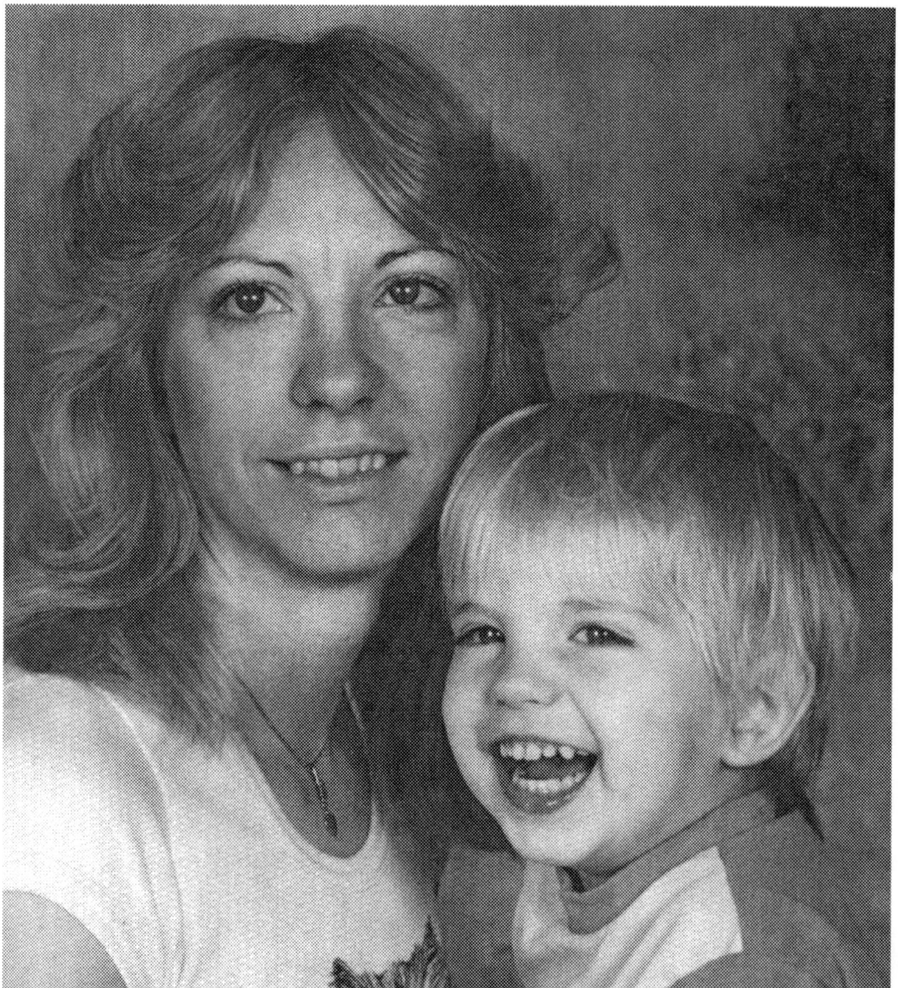

This Is a Story of Chad's Battle Through His Mother's Soul, Heart and Eyes

It had started out to be a typical hot, dry and windy June day in Kansas, just like every other Friday of my present life. Small town living with little to do seemed to get boring to me quite easily lately. It was the same routine day after day and seldom was there any excitement or change. Often I longed for something out of the ordinary to bring about some change, some excitement, some adventure, anything. I had no idea that on this day there would be a change that would be the beginning of one of my worst fears becoming a reality.

I was awakened at five-thirty in the morning by the high-pitch beeping of the alarm clock. Preparing for the day I was out the door to be at work by seven to start my day as usual. Soon it was finally time to go home for lunch. As I was getting ready to walk out the front door of the house to return to work something inside my brain urged me to check the answering machine on the phone, something I seldom did at lunchtime. The light was flashing on the caller ID. Pressing the button I heard my son's voice saying, "Mom, you need to call me back as soon as you get this call."

Hearing fear and a tremor in my son's voice I knew it was not good news. My thoughts were that he or his fiancée had been in a traffic accident where they lived in Atlanta, Georgia. With him and his fiancée living in such a big city I always was concerned of them driving in the traffic.

I quickly picked up the phone and placed the call that would travel one-thousand fifty miles of wire in seconds. Thank goodness for the invention of the telephone. I was relieved to hear his voice say "Hello" as he answered the phone. I knew that meant he was okay so my concern went to if something had happened to Rachael, his fiancée. I inquired of him what was going on and if he and Rachael were both okay.

Upon my son's response I felt my legs become as rubber and do not know how I was still standing as they continued to hold me up. I heard these sobbing words, "Mom, they said I have leukemia. I need you out here as soon as possible."

Somehow I managed to speak as I sat down on the edge of the recliner in the living room. I reassured him that I would be there as quickly as I could and would start making arrangements for a flight from Kansas to Georgia immediately.

My first thoughts in making the return call were that there had been an accident and he and/or his fiancée were injured. Never in my wildest dreams or imagination did I think it was going to be news that my son had a deadly disease that was killing him. He had always been healthy and strong. No one in our family had any history of cancer so the thought had never crossed my mind.

My thoughts drifted to picturing where he told me he was at the present time. There was my son, at age twenty-four, lying on a hospital gurney and was going to be taken for a bone marrow biopsy. He was taken directly over to the hospital from his doctor appointment for admission. The doctor would not even let him return home for personal items. The hospital staff was quickly starting preparations for him for a long hospital stay. There seemed to be a big sense of urgency in his care. I cringed in thinking of the fear he was going through. My heart ached for him. I was sure he felt scared, helpless and alone in the world at that very moment.

Here was a young man who had left work and gone for an appointment to see the doctor that day for a sinus infection. He was expecting to return to work and then go home to his normal routine. Now he had just found out he was dying. He had become a prisoner to a form of blood cancer with little hope even for parole.

There lay my son one-thousand fifty miles away from me in Atlanta, Georgia, scared and hurting. His fiancée was by his side but there was no other family or friends living even close. The two had only moved to Atlanta six months before this life-threatening news came to us. With settling into their new home, environment and jobs, there had not been much time for socializing and making new friends.

I quickly tried to give him reassuring words that all would be okay and I would be there as quickly as I could. I felt scared and my head was spinning as I hung up the phone and sobbed my heart out and prayed.

One cannot describe what a parent feels at that very second in time. Feelings of fear, anxiety, denial, confusion and anger were going through me all at the same time. No parent wants to lose a child to death. No child is supposed to die before the parent. In my mind I traced the time from my conception of him to the present time as a flash on a movie screen. I was searching and wondering if it was something I had done in raising him that had caused this ugly illness to be in him.

I had been raising him as a single parent since he was ten and his younger brother at age five. My two sons were the center of my universe and losing them was a fear I had carried inside me ever since they were babies. I recalled how Shawn, my youngest son, had almost been kidnapped before he was even two. I recalled how it was difficult to see Chad grow up and move so far away and knew Shawn would someday possibly be doing the same.

As they were growing up I could always make things better when they were hurt, both physically and emotionally. I knew in my heart that this time I could not "kiss it and make it better" or cover it up with a bandage. I knew I could not keep telling him everything was going to be okay, even though I had just told him it would be over the phone. I felt totally helpless. There was no bandage big enough that was able to cover this hurt.

I knew I would have to go inform his younger brother of what I had just learned. Growing up over the years the boys had become each other's best friend. They shared so many special times together and the brotherly love between them put a bond between them. Trying to figure out what I was going to say and how I was going to say it played heavy on my mind as I drove to Shawn's house. How was I going to tell an eighteen-year-old that his only brother is dying?

I had departed from my house quickly but slowed the car down with each block closer to his house. I pulled up into the driveway and parked the car in front of his house. I sat there for a few minutes just staring at his front door. Shawn was on the other side of that front door with no idea that the news that he was about to receive was going to tear his world to shreds. I wondered how he was going to handle it emotionally and how he would react.

Wiping my tears from my face and taking a deep breath I got out of the car and walked to the front door. There were still no easy or comforting words that were coming to my mind even as I knocked on his door. My stomach was in knots and my head throbbed as I heard my youngest son unlocking the front door. I now felt my heart aching terribly for both my sons.

I had worked on an oncology ward in past years with people having cancer and knew that the outcome for Chad may not be good. I knew the odds were against him. I had seen the fear and pain in a cancer victim's eyes. I had seen the pain and helplessness in their families. I had talked to them and their families but somehow this was different. It was my family and my child. I tried to recall how the doctors seemed to inform the patient and their family so easily that they had cancer. It was useless to me right now. Never had I ever considered the fact that the ugliness of cancer would present itself into my family.

There was only the three of us in our little family for the past fourteen years and we could not afford to lose one. Chad was the living flesh I had given birth to. He was a part of me. A part of me that was now dying.

Shawn opened the door. Upon entering the living room I told Shawn that he needed to sit down. At that moment he knew I was not there to give him good news by the look on my face and the tone in my voice. He could see the worry on my face, hear the fear in my voice, and see that I had been crying. He thought it was going to be bad news about one of his grandparents.

Before I spoke any further, I positioned myself on the edge of a chair that was at an angle beside the one he had sat down in.

"What is it, Mom? What is wrong?" prompted Shawn.

I leaned forward towards him knowing that he was going to need to be held after hearing the news. All I could get out of my mouth was to tell him straight out that his only brother called and he was diagnosed with leukemia. I told him everything that I knew that Chad had told me. Through hard felt tears we held each other and cried mercifully. He immediately knew that we would be leaving quickly and that we were facing a long journey ahead. He also knew that we would be helping Chad fight this battle in every way we possibly could.

We spoke of how quickly we would need to leave and what he would need to do to prepare for this journey. Upon leaving Shawn's, he immediately began packing his suitcase and preparing for the unwelcome journey of a lifetime. I advised him that I would be calling him as each step was completed to take our journey.

Knowing we would both need added support, I contacted Tina who was my best friend and my sister-in-law to tell her of the latest news and see if she could get away from work on short notice. Since high school days Tina and I had always been there for each other for support through our hard times. We had shared laughter, joy, anger, tears, hurts, fears, and all emotions together. I knew I would need her and could count on her more than ever now. She and my brother, Danny, were like second parents to both my sons, as her two sons were to me.

If I were to need to stay in Georgia for a long period of time I did not want Shawn to have to make the journey back to Kansas by himself. He would be feeling such mixed emotions and have difficulty in leaving his brother's side. Also not knowing what we would encounter on our arrival it would be good to have her there. I did not know if we would even arrive on time in the event that he may pass away.

Tina informed me that she was pretty sure she would have to return to work within the next week but that she would check with her boss and call me back as soon as she found out if she could be off work.

An hour and a half had passed by quickly since I had taken off from work for lunch break. I knew I needed to return back to work to inform my boss as to why I had taken such a long lunch break. I would also need to explain to him that I would have to be gone for an undetermined amount of time. I had set in my mind that if being with Chad meant losing my job then that is what the cost would be. My mind was totally consumed and my body numb as I drove past familiar places but did not notice them on the short drive back to the office. The entire outside world had seemed to disappear from my sight and my mind.

I walked past everyone quickly as I went through the building to the boss's office. I did not want anyone to stop and ask me why I had been late. My red eyes were fixed straight ahead; I did not want anyone to see I had been crying. Entering the boss's office I slumped down in a chair across the desk from him. Fighting back the tears I informed him of the situation. I informed him that I was leaving work immediately and had no idea when I would return from the scene of the battlefield. He was very understanding. He permitted for a leave for as long as was needed. As I stepped back out of his office I could feel the whirlwind once again start around me. "I must get there as quickly as possible," I said to myself.

As I was driving back to the house to start packing I received a phone call from Shawn. He informed me that he had called his boss but his boss did not believe him when he told him of the situation. He thought Shawn was just making up a story to be off work. He was informed by his boss that if he did not report for work that evening he would be fired. As more time was used by delays I was becoming frustrated. I promptly turned the car towards Shawn's house to pick him up so we could go talk to his boss together. He was in no shape emotionally to be driving and I seemed to think I was.

I was angered as I entered the store where he worked. Why would they think that someone would make up such a horrible story to ask for time off? A short visit with his boss set things in order and Shawn would be off for the rest of the week and still have his job. We were also informed by his boss that he would have to return to work in four days or lose his job. I told them that it would depend on what the situation was when we got to Atlanta and I would inform him if Shawn needed to stay longer.

We were walking through the parking lot, leaving Shawn's place of work, when I received the most welcome call from Tina. Her boss had no problem with letting her get off work for such a family emergency. I felt a small twinge of relief deep down inside amongst the turmoil.

Upon returning Shawn back to his home, so he could finish preparing for our journey and packing, I drove back towards work to get plane tickets ready since I knew now how many to purchase. I had no computer at home. I returned to work and got approval from the boss to use the computer for getting on the internet to get airline tickets. Upon arriving back to the office I was approached by several co-workers. They had been informed by the boss of what had happened. Everyone was sympathetic and offered comforting words. It was nice to know I had such good friends and that they would be there to support me emotionally.

Never before had I trusted a computer with my credit card number, but this was an emergency and I would have to put my faith in the system. Connecting to the Internet I searched and found airline tickets for Shawn, Tina and me for a mere one-hundred thirteen dollars for each round-trip ticket. It was a very small amount to pay for the next day's flight. I was thankful for a little good luck for me in all the confusion. I booked our three round-trip tickets with the airlines, printed our itinerary and headed home to get out a suitcase and start packing. The three of us would be flying out the following morning. I prayed that that would be soon enough.

I knew I had to be in Atlanta by Monday, at the latest, as that is when they would start Chad's chemotherapy treatments. Chad requested that they not start the chemotherapy until I was there at his bedside. That reinforced to me the fear he was feeling. Realistically I knew I had to be there as soon as possible for emotional support for him and his only support system there, Rachael. I felt pretty sure that she was not handling the situation very well herself and that right now she felt pretty scared and alone also. I knew we needed to be there as soon as possible because we had no idea how long it would be or how close Chad was to death.

While finishing up loose ends of business that needed to be completed and packing a suitcase for a journey in fear, my fiancé returned home from work. I heard him come in and go into the kitchen. I had been in the bedroom so I proceeded to follow him into the kitchen. As I stood by the dining room table I told him of the news I had gotten and what all had taken place so far that day. He was standing across the room and was listening to my every word. Tears began to fall and I had to sit down on the dining room chair as I felt I was going to crumple to the floor. My legs once again became too weak to hold up my body. The comforting I was searching for in my heart did not prevail itself.

At some point and time that evening I just had to stop and gather my thoughts and feelings and go through my mental checklist to see if I had covered everything. It was so hard to concentrate. It was hard to understand why and how everyone and everything around me went through normal motions and activities. The world as I had known it was crumpling about my feet and no one seemed to notice.

Rachael called to let me know that the bone marrow biopsy went well, that Chad had been admitted to a room on the fifth floor of the hospital and that he was napping off some sedation. I informed her I would contact her again later that evening but to call me immediately if there were any changes or new updates. She seemed to be holding up very well emotionally by the tone of her voice. Yet I knew that a person responds differently when they are in a desperate situation than when it is calmed down and reality seems to present itself.

I went out to the backyard and sat down slowly in a lawn chair. Placing my hands over my face I cried and prayed desperately. I knew in my heart that there was nothing I could do to "make it go away" on my own. I had always been the strong one before this that could fix anything or somehow make it all better. That was not so this time. I wanted to scream, I wanted to run somewhere, because my mind and body were becoming more and more hysterical as I thought about the situation. I wished I could just pretend that none of this was happening. I wanted to smash or hit something in anger. But I knew the words I had heard earlier that day were real. I wanted to wish them away and I wanted to pretend I had not heard them. I wanted to be held and comforted. None of these things happened. I just sat there feeling numb and wept.

Facing reality, I asked God for a sign that Chad would be made well. Upon opening my eyes and looking up I saw a white butterfly fluttering around over the garden. I had always thought that seeing a white butterfly meant good luck. What I saw in my heart and thought in my mind was how a caterpillar goes into a cocoon and comes out a new beautiful butterfly. Chad would be in his cocoon (God's hands and angels' wings) for a while but then he would emerge from this as a better and stronger beautiful healthy person.

With anger I told Satan to be gone and quit confusing my thoughts and for God to help me with my faith to know that He answers prayers and would heal my son. I also felt the nagging ache in my heart from reality that many people die of cancer and that sometimes the answer to prayers is "no" if it is not in God's will. Fear returned to consume my body.

My mind drifted back to the month before when I had just been with Chad and Rachael for a week-long visit. I recalled how I almost did not make that trip. I recalled his feeling sick at that time with what we thought was a bad sinus infection. I recalled the wonderful memories we had made together during that visit. I realized now that he had leukemia then and it was taking over his body but we had no way of being aware of it. Cancer was not even an option we had considered for his not feeling well. I also realized how precious every moment of that week with him now was.

Chapter 2
May 2001

Hold Fast to the Memories

Material things do come and go
Some into the trash we throw
But memories last for a lifetime
And they do not even cost a dime

Memories are held inside
Made from the mountain peaks to the ocean's tide
Material things can soon be forgotten
And some of them even turn rotten

Make the memories when you get the chance
For everyone comes to the end of the dance
Those you hold so loving and dear
Their voice you may no longer hear

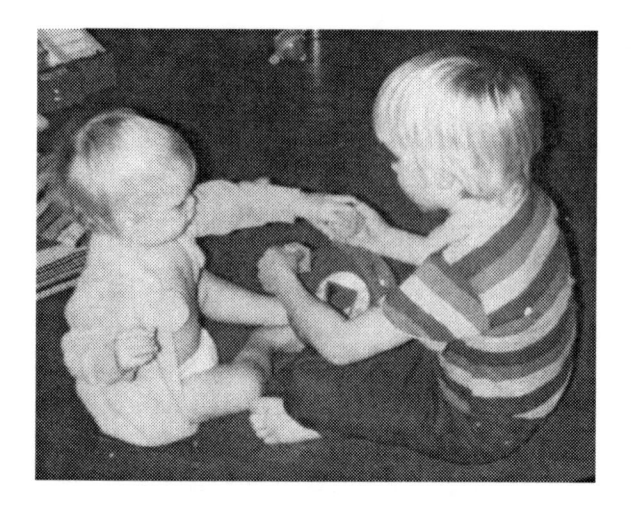

Big Brother Chad Teaches Little Brother Shawn

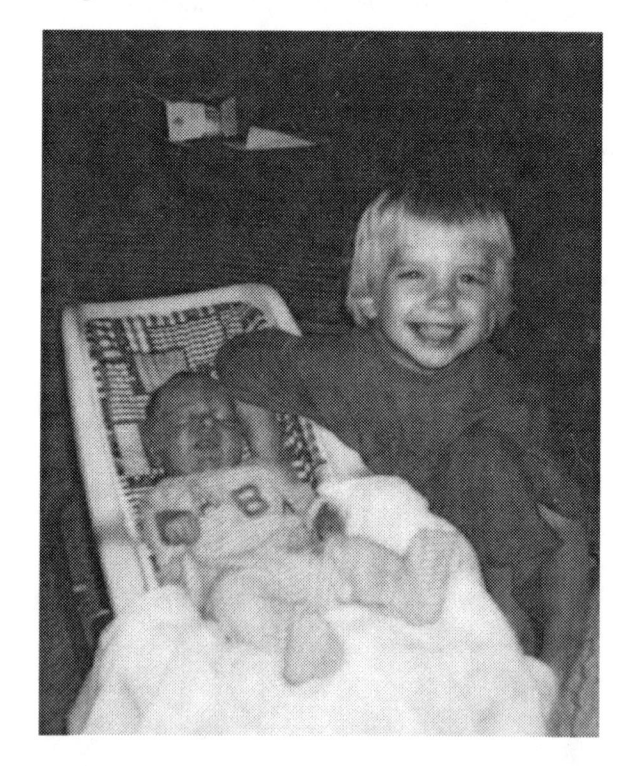

A Proud Big Brother to Shawn

It had only been four weeks before the frightening phone call in May that I had flown to Atlanta to have a week-long vacation with my oldest son, Chad and his fiancée, Rachael. It was a trip that I almost did not make.

At that time the airline prices were skyrocketing with it being the beginning of summer vacations and spring breakers. I had been watching airline prices for three weeks prior to the planned date of departure. I knew I could not spend a lot on an airline ticket so kept watching prices over that time.

I thought that the weekend I had told Chad and Rachael I would be there was on a three-day weekend from work but I had figured it wrong. I would have to use an extra day of vacation time. Since I had already committed that weekend to them I did not want them to have to change their schedules and plans around again. Both of them had already made arrangements to be off work for my visit. Prices of airline tickets continued to be around five-hundred dollars round-trip as I checked daily.

I finally felt defeated and thought I had better let them know that I would not be able to come out and see them financially. The day I was going to call to let them know I would not be visiting, the tickets were on the rise in price again. I kept stalling on making the call because I so deeply wanted to see them. During my lunch break I ventured to check one last time before I made the phone call to them. To my amazement the price of the ticket had dropped to two-hundred thirty-three dollars for the exact flight I had been watching. I called and booked myself on the flight instantly.

Just out of curiosity I looked up the price of the ticket at four that afternoon and it had risen to eight-hundred dollars. I thanked God for letting me find it at that price at the last minute so I would not have to cancel my trip. Pure luck on my part? I thought so at the time but looking back I now know that there was a reason God opened that little window one time over a three-week period for me to get that ticket. It was meant for me to go and see Chad. God was not ready for Chad to join him in Heaven; He still had plans for him on earth.

Chad and Rachael met me on my arrival at the Atlanta airport. They were a most welcome sight to see as I stepped off the plane. At that time visitors were able to go directly to the gate to meet passengers. We were anxious to see each other; it had been several months since the last time we had shared time together. When they picked me up Chad was not feeling well. He had the signs and symptoms of a bad sinus infection that he said had been going on for two weeks already. His sinuses were stopped up and he had a terrible headache that would not seem to go away. He had been trying everything he could find that was over-the-counter medications to take. Some things seemed to ease the pain a little but nothing made it go away.

Our plans were to go to Tybee Island but I suggested that we go to the beach another time since he felt so ill. He insisted that he felt well enough to continue with our plans to go and spend a couple of days at the beach. Chad loved the beach. He had always loved the water. At the age of six months I had taken him to water babies training. By the time he was twelve he was ready for lifeguard certification though he was too young to get it. He had been on the swim team during his school years. He had gotten to snorkel in the clear blue Caribbean waters and was only feet from a barracuda. One of his biggest joys was when I sent him birthday money so that he and Rachael could take scuba diving lessons in the past year.

We drove to the island and checked in at our hotel. It was evening by the time we got settled in but took a walk on the beach with flashlights in hand. Chad loved walking the beach at night to see what kind of treasures and interesting items the sea would place on the beach. He also loved to find the sand crabs and marveled in watching them run sideways.

After a night's sleep we were up and ready to greet the beach in the morning's light. Chad taught me how to boogie board on the waves and how to find sand dollars out in the ocean with my feet. We searched for seashells and relaxed on beach lounge chairs to let our bodies absorb the warmth of the sun. We climbed the stairs of the lighthouse. We walked amongst the large moss-covered oaks about the streets and squares of Savannah. We were talking and laughing all the while making wonderful memories.

For some reason Chad would frequently make jokes associating different things with a monkey to make us laugh. That entire weekend he seemed to be able to connect almost everything with a story about a monkey.

Chad showed joy in his face as he showed me the sights of the city's historical district. He seemed to be mesmerized by this city and wanted to share it all with me by showing me what all he had seen before. He acted as my private tour guide and joyfully told me all he had learned about Savannah and its history from his past visits. He spoke of the beauty he saw in the Tybee Island lighthouse and how it was his favorite lighthouse.

Excitement and energy was what was seen in his eyes but his body could not portray the same. He would tire easily and on occasion we would have to stop walking so he could sit and rest. We would sit down on the steps of a historical building or one of the many benches around town or in one of the peaceful squares so he could rest. Since Chad felt so badly, I felt bad that we had made this trip but the memories were priceless. Chad reinforced that even though he felt badly he was very glad we made the trip. Chad was determined when his mind was set on something.

Chad and Rachael were excited about getting me on a ghost tour, which Savannah is well known for. On our second evening at the beach we drove the twelve miles into Savannah from the beach hotel. We first strolled for a short walk down on River Street where we watched artists, performers, listened to street players and watched several huge ships come down the river. As it was starting to get dark we then took a ghost tour. Several times during the tour Chad would want to know what I thought of it all. He wanted this last evening in Savannah to be an exciting and memorable one. He accomplished his goal. The next morning we would be returning to Atlanta and Chad could get more rest.

Chad had been a real trooper all weekend and did not show how ill he really was or complain until our last morning there. Chad did not want to spoil our plans but he was ill enough that morning that he just wanted to stay in bed while Rachael and I walked the beach one more time before leaving the hotel. I knew by his actions that he was feeling worse.

Rachael and I did go beach combing after Chad reassured us he would be fine. He stayed in bed to get a little more rest. Someone had told us the previous day where a good place on the beach was to search for shells. We had not been over to that area of the beach before. We were gone a little longer than we had planned.

We parked in a small parking area and went for our walk. We did not think how each wooden walkway over the sand dunes looked just like the next. It took us a little more time finding the right one to cross over as we had walked farther on the beach than we realized. We did return to the hotel in time to load the car with our travel bags and check out.

Upon returning to the hotel we found Chad dressed and resting on the bed. He was still not feeling well. After checking out of the hotel we were on the road to return to Atlanta. Chad started out driving but after an hour had to give in to his illness. He could not make the entire four-hour drive back. He asked me to drive and I took over the driving so he could lie in the backseat. I drove until we were about thirty miles out of Atlanta. I was still not sure about driving through such a big city. Chad then took over the driving once again and drove us to their apartment.

I knew that Chad needed to see a doctor. I myself was prone to sinus infections and knew they could be very painful. All his complaints were similar to the symptoms I was familiar with. I knew that if Chad had an infection he would have to get antibiotics. It lay heavy on my heart to see him so ill.

The following day, Monday, I was going to be leaving so Chad and I had planned on doing a little shopping as I had a later flight in the day. Following what I was feeling in my heart I asked him to make an appointment to see a doctor before I left. His health had become a major priority and concern to me. I could not leave his side with him being ill and not getting treated. Reluctantly Chad agreed after I was persistent. Amazingly the doctor could see him that morning when he called to make the appointment. What a blessing. I was relieved. Instead of going to the mall to get me some new eyeglasses, I was more than glad to be going with him to an appointment with his doctor.

I packed my suitcases and loaded them into the back of Chad's little red car. By the time we finished at the doctor's office it would be time to get to the airport. Once the bags were loaded we left the house.

The doctor was very nice. He came out to the waiting area and introduced himself and took Chad back to the examining room. When the doctor had finished examining Chad, he came out to the lobby and introduced himself to me. The doctor informed me that it was a sinus infection and gum disease. I gave a sigh of relief. But then he continued to say that he was very concerned about the swollen glands he discovered in Chad's neck area. The doctor put him on antibiotics and antihistamines. He was also given instructions that he was to return in a week if the swelling was not gone from his neck or if he still felt ill. I breathed easier with relief however still concerned and a little worried. Even as a child, Chad had never had the mumps so I thought perhaps that was what the problem may be or that the infection had gotten into his glands.

From the doctor's office we went directly to the airport so I could catch my flight. I hated to leave seeing him feel so badly but knew I must. I was persistent about Chad doing the follow-up with the doctor even if he felt better in a week. He promised me that he would. We hugged, wiped back the tears and each said, "I love you." Then I walked away from him to walk to the terminal to catch the plane to go back to Kansas. The shoes on my feet felt as if they weighed a ton each with each step I took that departed me farther away from him. There was a nagging ache in my heart as I boarded the plane. As the plane ascended I had to fight back the tears. Something inside my head kept telling me I should not be leaving. There was a nagging ache in my stomach and heart that was getting stronger that seemed to be trying to make my feet turn my body around and walk back to Chad. Never before had I had such strong feelings like this when leaving either one of my sons.

Chad did have to return to the doctor a week later. He continued to feel badly with no relief from either one of his medications. He was given new prescriptions for different antibiotics and antihistamines. Chad's glands in his neck were still swollen. With this visit the doctor decided it best to get some lab work done also. It was fortunate for us that the lab technician that tested his blood had previously worked in a cancer clinic. She picked up on the signs of leukemia right away when looking at the lab specimens and notified the doctor of her suspicions immediately. Before the blood work results returned to the doctor's office he called Chad to have him see a specialist immediately.

The lab test results were faxed over to the specialist in oncology. We were told that on an average it would take up to two weeks to get the appointment. The oncologist took one look at the lab results and said he wanted to see Chad that very day. That is the day that I received the phone call that I would never forget.

I now realize that God does work in mysterious ways sometimes. He always has a plan that we cannot always see to start with. If I had not gone out to visit Chad previously he would not have gone to the doctor when he did. He wanted to wait another week or two to see if he got better on his own. God had just used me to help save my son before we even knew he had a killing disease.

Realizing my present surrounding in the backyard once again, I gathered my thoughts and returned back to the current situation we were facing. I took a deep breath and returned inside the house to make final arrangements before our departure for an unwanted journey the next morning. I prayed to God that He would give me the strength I needed for whatever we were about to encounter.

Chapter 3
June 2001

Why

I stand and look up to the sky
In wonderment and ask "Why?"
There are some things that I can see
And feel inside of what must be
Most answers I can reason out
Even with the slightest doubt
There are times I just do not understand
Changes You make with a touch of Your hand
In time I know that I will see
There is a plan God has for all, including me
But until then I wish I knew
And that He would give me just a little clue
I will try and do my best
To not be anxious and look for rest

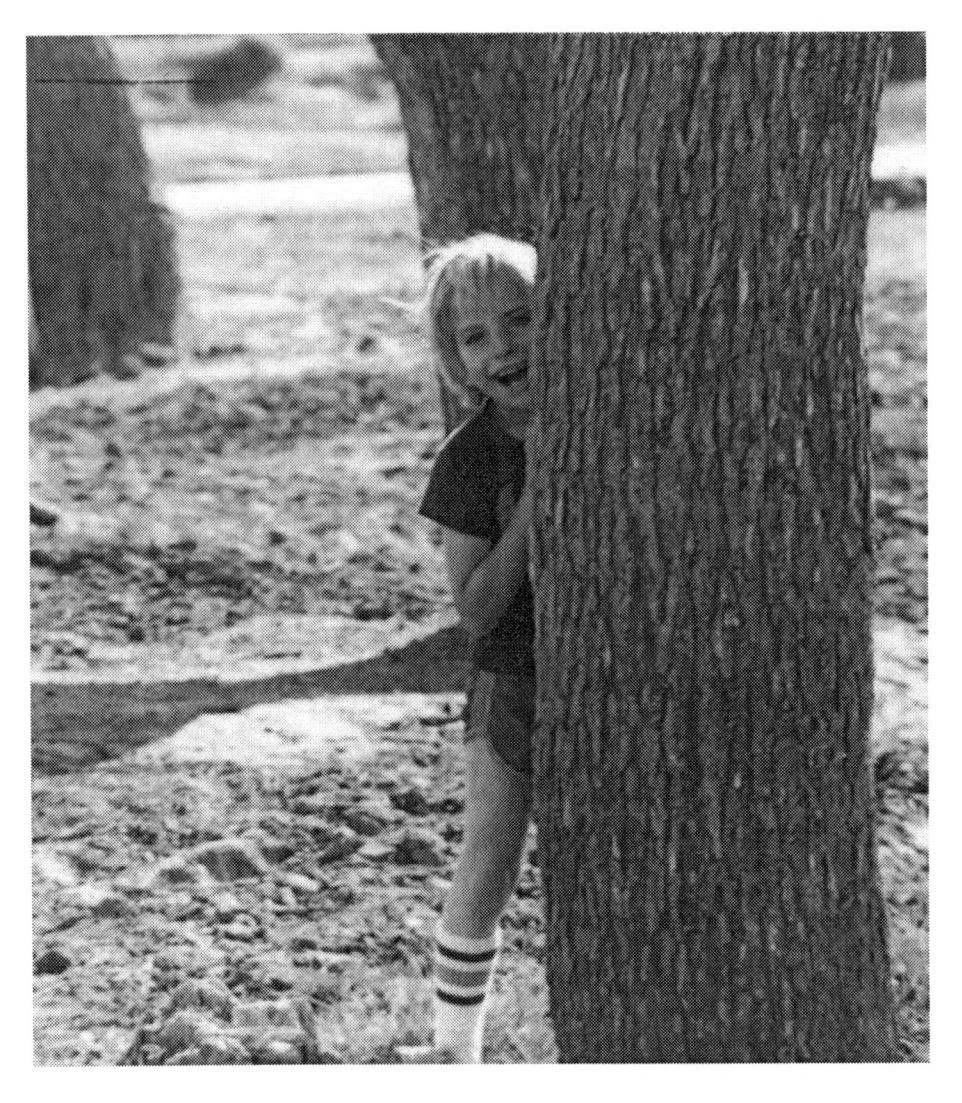

Now You See Me/Now You Don't
Today You See Me/Perhaps Tomorrow You Won't

Living in a small town in western Kansas, there are no large airports even remotely close. Shawn, Tina and I would have to make a five-hour road trip to get to an airport for a two-hour flight to Atlanta.

The next thing on my list of things to get done was to find a way to and from the airport. I did not want to pay to leave a vehicle at the airport because I had no idea how long I would be gone. Making phone calls I got arrangements made between my cousin Raina, my nephew Joshua and his wife Melissa and all was set. Raina would take Shawn and me to meet Tina at Joshua and Melissa's house in Wamego. My nephew would take the three of us to the airport in Kansas City, Missouri. They were more than glad to help out in a time of need. I was more than grateful to them. Another problem taken care of.

My two nephews, Jeremy and Joshua, had grown up with Chad and Shawn and all four boys were more like brothers than cousins. The four boys had grown up together and shared many experiences and made wonderful childhood memories. They were like my own sons as my sons were to Tina and Danny. They too were taking the news hard and wanted to do all that they could to help in any way possible.

I was pretty sure I had everything taken care of now and it was very late in the evening. I was emotionally exhausted and ready to try and get some rest for the next day's adventure to the unknown fearful territory. Atlanta had become our battleground and leukemia our enemy. It would be a fight to the end, my son's end, if we lost.

Before I could rest I needed to hear Chad's voice one more time. I called the hospital room that he had been admitted to. It was good to hear him talking even if it was difficult for him. He was more emotionally drained than I was and the doctor had informed the nurses to give him a mild sedative for anxiety.

Chad informed me that he was upset because the doctor would not wait until Monday to start the chemotherapy as he had requested (because he wanted me there when they did). Instead it had been started that evening. I would later find out how urgent the situation was. I reinforced to him that Shawn, Tina and I would be there the next day and I had a big hug waiting for him. I tried my best to keep a positive tone in my voice as not to show my fear and heartache. I was trying to convince him that it was going to be fine. By the end of our conversation he seemed to have a glimpse of excitement in his voice. As I sensed the fear he was feeling it overrode all the emotions I had been going through.

Preparing for bed I lay down in the darkness. The world seemed darker that night than it ever had before. The air felt cool and the silence more lonely than it had ever been in my life. Sleep did not come easily. Eventually I dozed off for a short time.

Saturday morning there was no ceiling on the anxiety I was feeling. I arose early and finished up anything I had thought of during my restless night to finish up. I checked frequently at the time awaiting the arrival of my transportation. Soon I saw Raina's car pull into the driveway. She had already gone by and picked up Shawn. Their arrival came all too soon in my mind as I proceeded out the front door. I was pretending in my mind that as long as I stayed inside this all would be a dream but the moment I stepped outside to start this journey I would be in another world. Reality and anxiety struck me hard as I got in Raina's car for us to depart.

All went as planned to transfer us from one place to the next to reach our final destination at the airport. Raina delivered us to Joshua and Melissa's house where we met Tina. Joshua and Melissa drove us to the airport for our departure. It was a long ride and I was glad to finally be at the airport because that meant we were only a few hours away from our landing time in Atlanta.

Once at the airport I felt a little less anxious as I knew we would be with Chad in just three hours and I had Shawn and Tina by my side. I always had more strength when I was with others. I tend to think that I need to be the strong one for everyone. I called Chad to see how he was doing and reinforced my love for him and to inform him that I would be there with him very soon. I was thankful he had made it through the night. I had also called Rachael earlier that morning to see how things were at the hospital. At that time Chad was sleeping and I did not want him awakened.

As the plane descended into Atlanta airport the nausea and knot in my stomach subsided some as well did my headache. Conversation between the three of us was general. None of us wanted to talk about the situation we were headed for. Rachael's boss met us at the airport. She had never met us before so was holding up a sign with my name on it. At some point many of us think how important we would feel to step off an airplane and have someone holding up a sign with our name on it. Not this time. We were too anxious and in too much of a hurry to even care. She felt our anxiety to get to the hospital and she promptly wasted no time in helping us get our bags and making our way quickly out of the airport.

It is difficult to say what all the three of us were feeling at that moment when we pulled up in front of the hospital. I know that fear was abounding in all of us. Fear of the unexpected, fear of losing Chad, fear that we may find he had already passed on, fear of seeing him so ill.

The hospital was such a massive big brick building and my son was somewhere inside waiting for me. We quickly departed from the car and entered through the two sets of large sliding glass doors. The marble floor seemed cold and uncaring as we walked to the cold steel elevator that ascended us to the fifth floor. Stepping off the elevator I took a deep breath and looked to see what direction to go for the room that was containing my son. We walked down the hall to Chad's room. Already fighting back tears I lightly tapped on the door then slowly opened it to Chad's room to step in.

As I opened the large wooden door to his room I could see the foot of the metal hospital bed. The tile was like all hospital tile, off white in color in squares on the floor. The walls painted the standard white with a television attached to the wall in the corner of the ceiling. It seemed so cold and lonely and brought reality to the whole situation. There were intravenous bags (IV) hanging from a portable stand that stood by the bedside running through a pump with tubes leading into Chad's body.

Rachael was sitting in a chair in the corner of the room by the head of the bed. Chad lay against the white sheets almost as pale as they were. He wore a white hospital gown with some type of small blue design on it which seemed to be the only color in the room.

I dropped my purse in a chair and quickly stepped to my son's bedside. He opened his eyes and looked at me and we held each other. Kissing him on the forehead, I told him "I love you." It was difficult to fight back the tears and not cry. I thought I needed to appear to be the strong one—to not show the true fear and heartache that was overwhelming my body and mind. I felt that if he saw me cry that it would give him more despair and fear that he was not going to pull through this. I felt that I must keep a positive outlook and tone of speech for him.

I knew at that moment that these four walls would become my permanent home for as long as need be because I was not leaving his side. It seemed to be uplifting to Chad to have Shawn and Tina come with me to his side. Yet his mind seemed to fade in and out of awareness. Part of this was due to the chemotherapy and part from the mild sedation he was receiving. Chad said his mind seemed to be in a different world at times and he felt this was all like a dream.

After a long day it was time for Shawn, Tina and Rachael to leave for the evening. I refused to budge from my son's side. I had brought him into this world and I was going to do all I could to help keep him in it. I removed my suitcase from Rachael's boss's car and Shawn and I said goodnight to the others. We held each other for several moments tightly before letting go.

Once all was quiet and it was just Chad and me, he wanted to talk. It was the hardest conversation I have ever had with anyone in my life. He and his fiancée were to be married that fall but he had decided to postpone the wedding. He informed me that he did not want to take the chance of making Rachael a bride and a widow all in the same year. He also talked of life insurance and burial. He was doing better at facing the possible end of this battle than I was. I told him that we would not continue the conversation unless it came to a time when it was really necessary. We talked of positive thinking and of faith in God.

I made a bed out of the chair in his room and we both slept for a short time. Sometime during that night I awoke to hear him crying. Going over to his bed I sat on the side and asked him what was wrong. He sat up and looked me straight in the eyes. His response was "I don't want to die."

We both knew that was a possibility of leukemia. I never believed in telling my children lies so I could not tell him that everything was going to be okay because I myself did not know for sure. I do know that I have never felt more helpless in my life before that time. Troubles I thought I had in the past were nothing now. I reassured him that I would be there for him. I spoke of how he would not be alone in this battle and that I would be there for him through it all. Reality was hard to face but we both knew we would face it side by side. Desperately I wanted to tell him that everything would be okay.

Once Chad seemed to be resting quietly again I settle back into the chair bed at his bedside. My mind drifted after our conversation and I wondered what Shawn was feeling. The two boys had always been very close. We were a strong family of three. I wondered how Tina was taking all this and thankful for her presence. I wondered how Rachael was holding up after having to face these last two days without support or someone to talk to. I was pretty sure that I was not the only one weeping tears of a heavy heart that night.

The following day I went down to the gift shop while Chad was napping. Since Chad was not allowed to have flowers in his room I thought perhaps balloons to cheer up his room and add some color would be helpful. Upon entering the hospital gift shop I spotted a large, hairy black monkey sitting on a shelf. It was the perfect gift. After purchasing it I took it up and placed it on the foot of Chad's bed for him to see when he woke up from his sleep.

Upon his waking he did not notice it right away. As he seemed to slowly comprehend his surroundings he spotted it. He laughed and a smile of joy came across his face. He once again started with the monkey jokes and was pleased to have this new "bed buddy."

The day was spent visiting and giving encouraging words. Tina filled him in on what had all been going on with Danny, Jeremy and Debi, Lane, Joshua and Melissa and other family members. Chad and Shawn spoke of friends that they had in common and recalled events of their childhood. It was a joy to my ears and my heart to hear Chad's laughter and see his spry outlook on life start to return.

That night Tina offered to stay during the night at the hospital, encouraging me to go to the apartment and get some rest. I knew she was well capable of helping care for Chad's needs but I could not get myself to depart his side. I would not even consider it. I had told Chad I would be there by his side through it all.

All too soon the four days passed and I lost the closeness of my two supporters. Shawn and Tina flew back to Kansas so they could both return to work and report back to family and friends. I promised to give them daily updates on what was going on. Now it was just Chad, Rachael and me to keep this battle going. There was much support and prayers being sent over the miles but it just was not the same as having a real person with you.

Because I wanted to be the strong one I refused to show or express my fears or speak negatively about the situation. I had always been a positive thinker and needed to lean on that concept heavily now. I feared that Rachael was doing the same thing, as she did not talk about her feelings to me either. She had lost her mother in her early teens in a hospital room so I knew it was a situation that would cause her anxiety. At times it seemed to me that she just avoided the situation and pretended that it was not happening. We all deal with things in our own way to get through them. What was she thinking I wondered to myself? Yet I did not ask. I was afraid that if we talked about it I would let down my "bravery" guard and my emotions would get the best of me and I would not be the strong one anymore. It would possibly force me to face the fact that my son may die.

During the first seven days in the hospital, Chad received chemotherapy. I still held on to some denial and fear that kept my insides churning. On the outside I portrayed the brave strong person. On the inside I was feeling the biggest fear-causing anguish a mother could have. I knew there were no promises, only hope, prayers and faith.

My heart ached as I watched the illness and chemotherapy start taking their course on Chad's body. The times of severe nausea, stomach pain, restless sleep, emotional tension and loss of appetite seemed to get worse with each passing day for Chad. The medications, intravenous fluids, lab work, shots and treatments seemed to be never ending as each day went by. Most of the time Chad spent trying to sleep and fight off the pain and vomiting. Almost daily he thanked me several times for being there. Just to have someone at the bedside was comforting to him. When one fears death I think one also fears dying alone.

We spent our time talking and keeping up with all the latest news about family and friends that were adding him to the prayer chain. There were people from Texas, Oregon, California, Alaska, Missouri, New York, Kansas, Florida, United Kingdom, Nebraska, Oklahoma and God only knows where all else as the chain grew. By use of e-mail, word spread near and far. I had been given permission to use the hospital library computers to check my email, send out updates and do research.

The youngest of prayers, to my knowledge, was from my great nephew, Lane. Jeremy called, as he often did, to see how things were going with Chad. On one particular phone conversation we talked of all the prayers that were going up to Heaven for Chad. Jeremy informed me that his five-year-old son, Lane, had surprised him at the supper table one evening. Lane asked if he could give the blessing before their meal. Jeremy was proud to hear him make his request. Lane started his prayer with a request to God to make Chad better. It was heartwarming to hear of this wonderful thing that a five-year-old wanted to do on his own accord. Jeremy also informed me that on that day Lane started adding Chad to his bedtime prayers.

As the prayer chain grew day by day, so did my faith. I decided that some of those people must be praying for me too as I felt stronger to face the situation. As Chad awoke alive each morning it gave us new hope for a day closer to possible remission.

One day I told Chad that I could visualize a mountain removed that was in front of him; because of prayers and faith the road was opened. I also prayed often for those who were praying for us. I thought of how it speaks in the Bible about the faith of a mustard seed moving a mountain. I decided that once I felt I could part from the hospital I was going to start looking for a mustard seed necklace. I had had one once as a child but it was so scratched up that you could not even tell there was anything in it. I was not sure that I even had it anymore. I continued searching each chance I got and over time I found one.

Two days had passed since the last of the chemotherapy treatments and things seemed to be smoothing out. The chemotherapy IV bags were now replaced with an occasional bag of blood or platelets.

That morning the doctor came into the room to inform us that the blood they had drawn earlier that morning had shown that there were no cancer cells left in Chad's bloodstream at that time. We breathed a deep breath of joy. Chad and I looked each other in the face with tear-filled eyes of happiness. We hugged and I felt I never wanted to let go.

Next would be another bone marrow biopsy to see if the bone marrow was also clean of cancer cells. There would be a two-day wait to get results from this procedure. It would seem like the longest two days of a lifetime. Usually it took from a week and a half to two weeks to get the results back but the doctor put a rush on it so that he could get the results as quickly as possible.

Since we had finally gotten good news I was able to read the literature that we had received from the hospital and the Leukemia Society regarding acute myelogenous leukemia. In it I read that the prognosis for this type of cancer was two months. I realized even more how powerful prayers and faith could be. It made me realize just how close to death my son had just been; it was scary to think of it in this way. The information I found in the literature gave me general insight as to the illness and its general effects but nothing about the small details of all the side effects and how to deal with the emotions.

The doctor and Chad reinforced the reality of my fear I had been feeling when they informed me that the reason the chemotherapy was started on Friday night instead of Monday morning was because if they had waited those two days Chad would have bled to death internally and would not have been alive that very day! My heart felt as if it was in my throat as I fought back more tears. I thought of how unselfish it was of Chad to think of how it would have made me feel if he would have told me this over the phone during our conversations before my arrival.

Waiting those two days for the biopsy results was stressful although we felt that if the blood work came back clean that the biopsy would too. We waited on pins and needles on that second day as the hours ticked by so slowly while we waited for the doctor to come into the room. I was beginning to feel that the results were not going to be good and therefore the doctor was delaying his visit because he did not want to tell us bad news.

As I thought about all Chad had before him and all that he could be and wanted to do, I prayed and drew on my faith until I just knew that the results were going to be good. The doctor finally arrived late that afternoon to tell us it was good news. The bone marrow biopsy was clean except for a couple of cancer cells but that it looked like they were dying. The pathologist had to hunt hard to find them.

For the second time in the two and one half weeks I had been there I went to Chad and Rachael's apartment to take a breather, do laundry and repack for the next week's hospital stay.

For the first time since Chad became ill we all finally felt some peace and calm inside us. A good deep night's sleep came most welcomed to each one of us that night. Before I fell asleep I felt the battle was won, only to find out later that the battle would still continue for some time.

Chapter 4
July 2001

Change of Life Purpose

When you grew up you wanted to be
A pilot with open skies to see
A bike racer to go for speed
A scuba diver to rescue those in need

I said you can be anything you want to be
Giving you hopes, dreams and encouragement was the key
I thought of you upon a stage
Your wit and humor being all the rage

You had dreams of college days
Walking the beaches in the sun's rays
Raising a family to love and to hold
Collecting things more precious than gold

All too soon your dreams had to change
New goals were now placed in your range
God changed your purpose to fight death in strife
He made you a brave hero in this life

HOLDING ON FOR DEAR LIFE

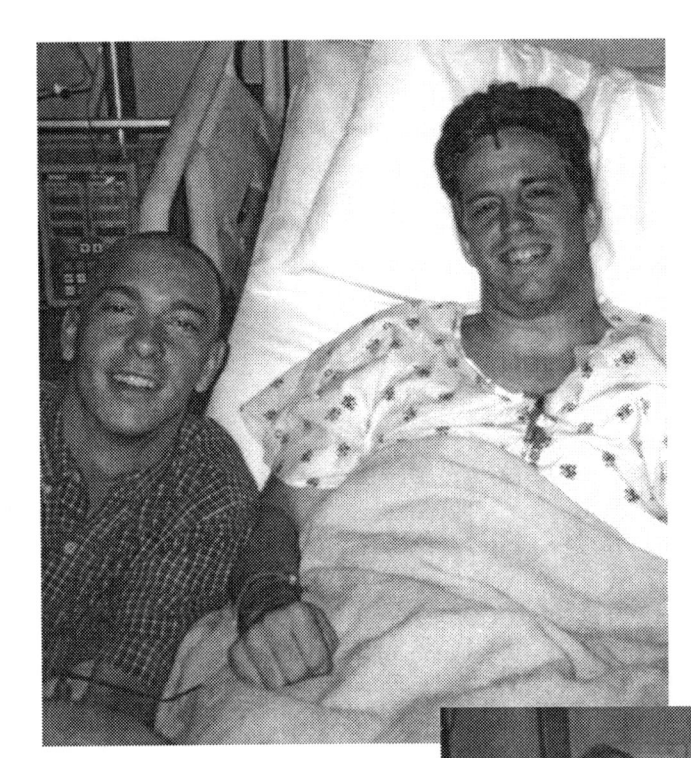

Shawn with Chad in Hospital

Aunt Tina with Chad in Hospital

Chad became neutropenic in the week to follow. This meant that he had absolutely no immune system. I was informed that even a simple cold could kill him. Now all his blood counts were gone, both bad and good. The risk of infection became a reality when the doctor told me that they lose more neutropenic cancer patients because of their being unable to fight against infections than from the actual cancer itself.

New fear and anxiety set in. I wished we had been aware of this before. But then there was really no choice. If they had not done the chemotherapy we would be putting Chad in his grave for sure. With the chemotherapy he at least ended up with a fighting chance. I wish we had known beforehand so that we could have at least prepared ourselves mentally for it, if that was possible. The leukemia cells were now a battle won but I had not been told previously that the treatment would cause him to have no immune system and the reality of death was still just as predominate as ever.

I became stressful because I was prone to sinus infections. What if I gave him an infection that would end his life? "God, keep me well and get his blood counts up to normal quickly," I prayed. If I even felt like I was having any physical problems of any kind I would take my temperature and wear a mask while around Chad. Hand washing was a must after touching almost anything. I was not sure I could bear to live with myself if I would cause him to die.

Being neutropenic came with more precautions. Chad was not to be near fresh fruits or vegetables, plants or any object with standing water. He was not to be anywhere that there was a crowd of people, was not to be near any children under the age of ten or anyone that may be ill. I was also informed that the chemotherapy canceled out any childhood immunity that he had received. This added to the fear of mumps, measles, and other communicable diseases that he could come into contact with. It would be doubtful that he would be in contact with anyone having a disease since he was in the hospital; there was always the chance that someone he would come into contact with, even a hospital employee could be a carrier. Rachael's job was a concern as she worked with small children. She had to be extremely careful.

These diseases would be certain death for him. If he was outside of his hospital room he had to wear a mask. Outside of his room he did not touch anything. I was the contact for all doorknobs, etc. No one was supposed to come near him if they had any signs at all that they even might be ill.

Good hand washing techniques were now a matter of life and possible death. I would watch anyone entering the room like a hawk for its prey to make sure everyone used the precautions and washed their hands and wore gloves for certain procedures. Our contact with the world was now at an extreme minimum. I only left the room when necessary. I did not want me or anyone else to become a carrier of any illness.

Chad's temperature had to be taken every four hours around the clock. If he started running a fever it would be every two hours. Now he would be more isolated from the world than ever. It was already becoming difficult for him to be as alone as he was such a person that loved to be around people. He started making more conversation with the nursing staff when they would enter his room. He started showing signs of becoming restless and bored but yet did not feel up to doing any reading, puzzles, etc.

The weeks were long and I quickly learned what it meant to have patience. It had always been difficult for me to sit still for very long, but I was now learning to do so. I would get out of the room and out of the hospital for short times on occasion when Chad was sleeping. At least I could walk around the hospital grounds and escape the four walls that surrounded our world, as we now knew it. It was not easy for Chad; he could not escape. He continued to be entrapped within those four walls facing the ever possible feared outcome.

I contacted a friend of several years that has the ability of what some people refer to as being psychic. I told him of the situation and concerns. He told me not to worry that everything was going to be fine. He talked to me at long length several times and helped to ease my mind and fears. In the past he had always been at least ninety-five to one hundred percent right on what he told me. Some people may think this a wrong thing to do but desperate times call for desperate measures if you see it that way.

He was now verbally complaining for the first time of being bored and was becoming depressed. Eating still remained a problem. Just the smell of food would bring about nausea to him. Rachael and I were allowed to bring in food from outside the hospital and would go get anything promptly that he was hungry for. There was a cafeteria and a snack bar in the basement of the hospital and several fast food places within two blocks walking distance of the hospital. When his hunger struck I had to move quickly, for if I were to wait he would not be hungry anymore. Even at that there were times I did not make it back quickly enough before the nausea started up again and the hunger left. Rachael would bring in anything she thought he might like to eat from home. Chad always welcomed her home-cooked meals and would voice his appreciation.

Impatiently we waited in the hospital for another two and one half weeks for Chad's white blood count to reach fifteen hundred from zero. Finally he was well on his way to a returning immune system. Normal range was from four thousand to ten thousand. As the blood count rose he had begun to start feeling better.

The doctor came into the room for his daily visit and began talking of releasing Chad from the hospital to go home. His blood counts had not totally reached the range that he was not neutropenic but the depression was becoming a concern.

The next day his white blood count dropped to four hundred. What was going on? Even the doctors could not explain it. Just as we started getting excited about the white blood counts coming up we became confused and upset when they dropped more two days later. The doctor started Chad on shots to help encourage the white cell counts to multiply faster, this in hopes of bringing his white count back up faster. Waiting it out with each day's blood draw results and the shots was aggravating to Chad. Finally the count slowly started coming back up again.

Once Chad's counts were steadily on an uphill climb the doctor allowed Chad to take short walks outside around the hospital as long as he would wear double gowns and a mask. It helped with the depression that was setting in for him to get out into the fresh air and sunshine. This unfortunately came to an abrupt halt after the second day that we took a walk. We were out walking one evening and passed by some bushes alongside the hospital. All at once he reached his left hand over to his right arm. He had gotten a bug bite on his forearm. Neither of us had thought of that possibility. We quickly returned to his room and informed the nurses. The area was cleansed and dressed and we kept a close eye on it. It went away without physical problems but caused Chad emotional worry.

Our Fourth of July celebration came and went with little to celebrate in the hospital. We were ungrateful because Chad had been given such a burden to bear but yet could celebrate his still being alive, right? That was not a task taken lightly or to be done as easily as it sounded. Chad was tired of the entire ordeal and wanted to go home. Even with him in remission from cancer he was far from being able to celebrate independence from this battle.

I had learned from the nursing staff of a race that was held every Fourth of July in Atlanta. They told me that the runners went on the road right in front of the hospital. The hospital was located only blocks from downtown. I went outside to watch for a short time as Chad watched for a few minutes from his room window. That evening Chad, Rachael and I looked out of his room window at what fireworks we could see flashing over Atlanta. It was difficult to see any so we got a chair and placed it at the end of the long hallway for Chad to sit in. He, Rachael and I watched at the fifth floor window at the end of the hallway of the hospital corridor to see the Fourth of July fireworks as best we could see them through the maze of treetops and downtown buildings.

After thirty-two days in the hospital Chad's blood count finally was back up to fifteen hundred. The doctor said he would send him home still neutropenic. He had been living within those four walls all too long. The depression was starting to leave its mark. We were given strict guidelines to follow for the next several weeks. Rachael cleaned the house thoroughly and cleared away all houseplants, as he still barely had any immune system.

Chad was thrilled at the doctor's words and could not get ready to leave fast enough. To get back home to his own surroundings, own bed and see his boston terrier, Mattie, were uplifting to his spirits. I was anxious to take him home but yet frightened that something would go wrong and I would not get him back to the hospital in time and he would die on the way to the hospital. The doctor reassured us that he was only a phone call away, twenty-four hours a day.

I recalled the time when Chad was about twelve and we were moving to a different house. He complained of not feeling well so he lay on the couch as I unloaded the car. I had told him that I thought he was faking it so that he did not have to help with the move. I swallowed back my words as later that afternoon I took him to the emergency room to find out that he had to have surgery to get his appendix removed. It was that same year in the fall that I recall him getting an antibiotic from the doctor for an infection. He had an allergic reaction causing him difficulty breathing so I rushed him to the emergency room with fear of him dying on the way.

Chad's release from the hospital was the end of round one of the intense high aero-c chemotherapy. Now the decision had to be made as to if he wanted to continue with the chemotherapy regimen or to have a bone marrow transplant. We were told that the bone marrow transplant would have no back-up plan if it did not work. There would possibly be a second chance if the decision were for the chemotherapy. At least then there would be a back-up chance for remission with a bone marrow transplant if the chemotherapy did not work. Our options were simple.

Should we chance putting Chad through the chemotherapy that may only lead to also having to go through a bone marrow transplant or just do the transplant and take a chance? With either decision we would have to pray for the best. Of course our only other option was to do nothing but that left the possibility of the leukemia cells returning at almost a guarantee.

Chapter 5
July 2001

If I Go

I know in time we all will go away
Here on this earth we do not stay
You did your best and won the battle
The chains of leukemia you did rattle

If God's will is that you go
I know seeds of love you did sow
What would you leave behind
Thoughts of you that will be kind

If you leave you will also stay
You will never completely go away
There are things you will leave behind
Between hearts your love will bind

If you go, you leave for us each
Happy memories of you and the strength you did teach

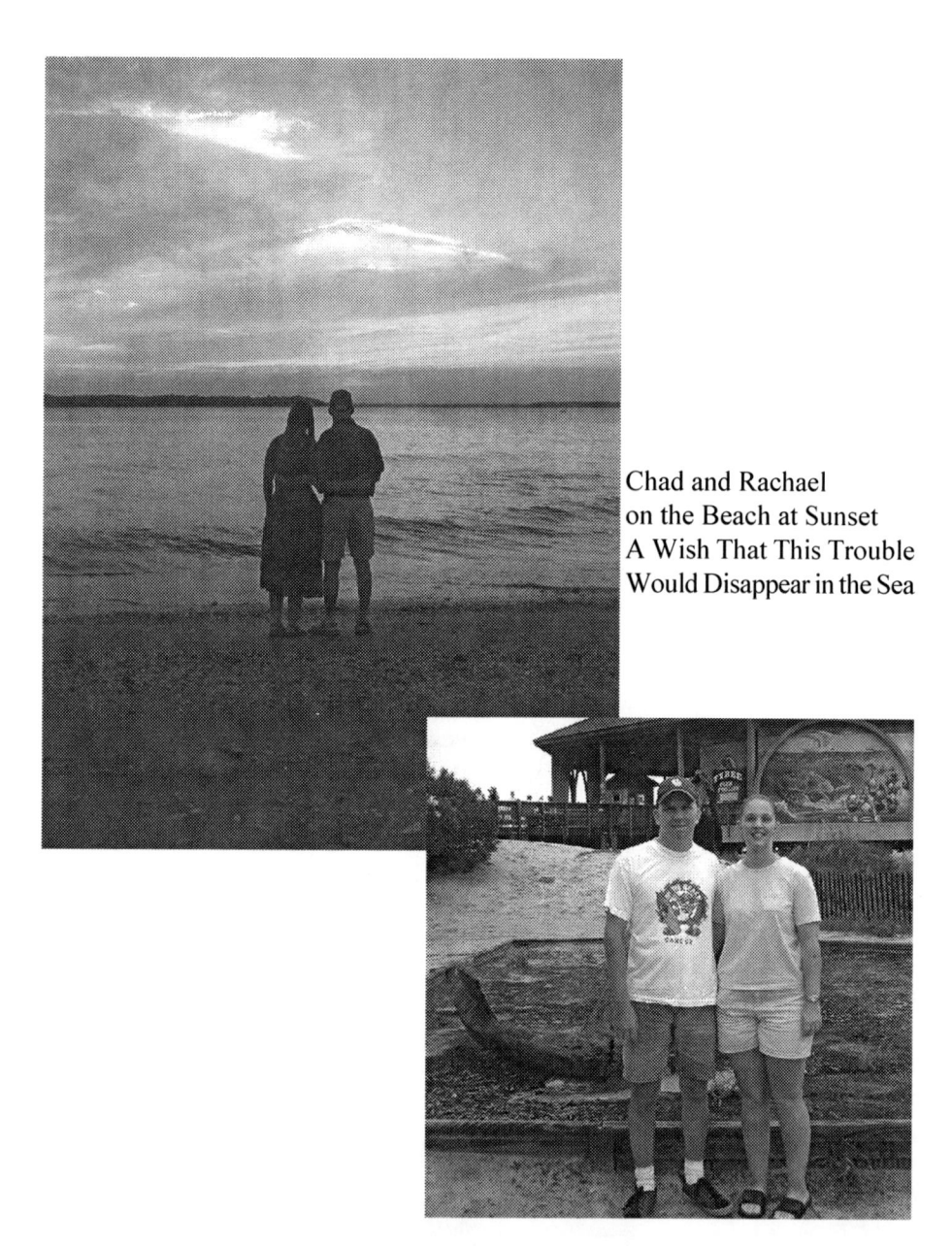

Chad and Rachael
on the Beach at Sunset
A Wish That This Trouble
Would Disappear in the Sea

I Will Love You Eternally

The doctor informed us that we could have up to two weeks to make a decision. He would set up an appointment for Chad to discuss the bone marrow transplant with a specialist to help him make his decision. The idea of possibly having a back-up plan gave me my decision; however, I wanted to let Chad make the final decision of what he wanted to do.

Even though Chad was doing well I was reluctant about getting a scheduled flight to return back to Kansas. I still feared for his life. His blood counts were still slow at progressing. The thought of something happening with me so far away again reinforced my fears and reluctance. It is amazing how the mind can work on you.

I knew financially that it was time to get back to work and to a now welcomed old boring routine for a little while. I packed my suitcase and flew back to Kansas. When I got back to work I tried to concentrate on work but thoughts of my son were overpowering most of the time. I almost constantly thought about the battle that lay before him no matter which decision he made.

We visited numerous times on the phone discussing the choices and possibilities. I told him of the pros and cons of both that I thought of. I let him know that he needed to make the final decision. I waited for his answer. The call finally came that let me know what his decision was for our next step in fighting this battle. He decided to try the chemotherapy regimen first. I agreed and told him that that is what I was hoping he would decide all along.

In just two short weeks the doctor placed Chad back into the hospital and started the second round of chemotherapy. Chad reassured me that I did not need to come be with him as he had been told that he would only be in the hospital a few days. They were going to administer the chemotherapy over a three-day stretch and then release him to go home. With him now in remission and thinking we were out of the danger zone, I decided not to return to be with him for his second treatment. Chad was now considered in remission and seemed to be holding out well emotionally.

I later found out that it was a wrong decision to make. Although we talked on the phone daily, he needed me there for emotional support but would not tell me. The nursing staff later told me that Chad would pull the covers up over his head and barely acknowledge anyone that came into the room. He did not want to watch television, read or talk to anyone. Due to financial obligations, Rachael could not stay with him as she had to continue working. She had no choice. I should have known when he had first called and told me that he was diagnosed with leukemia and that he needed me there that he needed me there for everything. I realized how much he needed me to lean on and to be his strength for him during the times of treatment and illness.

I also found out that the pain, nausea and vomiting were becoming overwhelming to him. I do not think that any of us thought it would be so intense.

During this time in the hospital the doctor also surgically put a port in his chest. This port was placed under the skin and would be used for insertion of his IV therapies. He would not have to be stabbed in the arm every time he needed an IV medication. Because of this port he would also be placed on a medication that would keep his blood thinned to hopefully keep any blood clots from forming that would clog up the port.

A new worry was now added. If Chad would get a cut or bruise badly he could bleed to death. It seemed that every few weeks that passed brought new concerns and fears. I did more research and asked more questions but still found nothing that told me of the details of the treatments. The doctor and nursing staff also chose not to volunteer all the "little" details that went along with going through chemotherapy. I am the type of person that would like to know all the information in the beginning and I was only getting it in pieces as I asked questions with any new event that Chad had happen to him.

While Chad was in the hospital the events of 9/11 took place. The terrorists placed planes into the World Trade Center. My conversations over the phone with Chad on this event were very emotional. It was hard for him to be lying in the hospital bed fighting with all he had to stay alive from a disease that was slowly trying to kill him. All the pain and suffering he was going through with the treatments was unimaginable to anyone that has never been through it. In his eyes those people went to work healthy and did not have to suffer for days on end as he was doing. Most of those victims saw instant death. He said he would rather opt for instant death than the slow agonizing death he felt he was facing.

This conversation made me wonder if he was going through all this pain and suffering because we wanted him to as an act of our own selfishness. I wondered if Chad really wanted to go through all this for himself. It was his nature to want to please others, to make life easier for them, and make them laugh so that they were enjoying their life. My heart continued to ache with the miles between us when we spoke over the phone.

Upon completion of the second round of chemotherapy he was released to go back home. He had to take his temperature every four hours and watch for any signs of infection due to the chemotherapy depleting his immune system once again. His counts once again dropped and he became neutropenic.

To all our fear he awoke one night to find he was running a fever and called the doctor. The doctor informed him that he needed to go to the emergency room to be admitted immediately. Chad drove himself to the hospital emergency room and was admitted. I received the call the next morning to let me know of the night's events that peaked my stress level again. I was concerned once again of possible infection. Knowing Chad, I was pretty sure that he had told Rachael to stay in bed and he would drive himself to the hospital. He never wanted to inconvenience anyone. The doctor and nursing staff were at awe that Chad had taken himself to the emergency room.

It was even harder now to concentrate on anything else in my world of chaos. My everyday routine picked up right where it had left off with little or no change. However, the emotional rollercoaster was almost more than I could handle. I realized that I had no control over the events and that I would have to pray for God to take care of him. Still I was constantly wondering how Chad was doing. I decided that I would not let him go through this alone again and made plans through my boss to be with Chad for the rest of the chemotherapy treatments.

For the next two weeks we continued to talk on the phone daily. Not only was my mind in Georgia but also was a big part of my heart. This caused me to have some guilt feelings as the other part of my heart was in Kansas. I knew I was also needed in Kansas to be there for Shawn.

At times I would call the nurses station to see how Chad was doing between the calls to him for fear of waking him if he were resting. Reassurance would always follow my conversations with him in hopes that it would uplift his spirits to continue his fight to live. With medications the doctor got the infection under control and after a two-week hospital stay Chad was released to return home once again.

I informed my boss that the chemotherapy treatments would be administered every four to six weeks depending on how long Chad would get past being neutropenic and I would need to be gone during those times. I was fortunate that they were willing to keep my position there for me at work. I knew I would be gone a lot over the next six months to a year. Even if it would have cost me my job, there was no way I would let Chad go through a chemotherapy treatment or hospital stay again by himself. I was not sure how bills were going to get paid but knew that God would somehow provide. I knew I would be living on faith and prayers.

All too soon I got the call that the third round of chemotherapy was to be started. It was not so much the fear of the chemotherapy that bothered me as it was the fact of the toll it took on Chad's body and mind during these treatments. It was also the reality that the effects that the chemotherapy would cause could possibly cause us to lose him. It seemed overwhelming at times. I could not get the doctor's words out of my head, "We lose more cancer patients from them being unable to fight off illness than from the cancer itself."

Chad was in remission but still had to go through all the chemotherapy treatments. I just could not comprehend why they just could not do chemotherapy treatments IF the leukemia came back. I understood that they wanted to make sure all the cancer cells were killed but at the same time I did not want to see my son go through such agony. Just as he was starting to feel better they would give him another round of chemotherapy that would knock him back down. I had to put trust in the doctor to do what was right. I prayed for God to guide the doctor in his decision making. I prayed for God to give Chad the strength and heal him.

Once again I found myself packing for the long haul. This time I drove to my niece Valerie's house just outside of Kansas City and would leave my car there. Valerie and I talked of the special relationship she and Chad had over the years. Chad was shorter than most boys his age until he got into high school. It had become a custom for he and Valerie to stand back to back on Christmas day to see who was the tallest. She was ahead for some time until Chad finally outgrew her and remained taller. The following morning Valerie took me to the airport. With heavy heart but anxious to see for myself how Chad was doing, I boarded the plane that would take me from Kansas City back to Atlanta. My emotions were running high. Chad had voiced his excitement of my return and calmness was in his tone when I told him I would soon be there for him once again.

It was a blessing to me to see Chad able to be at the airport when I got past the terminal gates. I had only expected to see Rachael. His body seemed fragile and his color pale but his smile was brilliant. Chad's attitude seemed to be a positive one. Once again he was handling all of this better than me. I hoped that knowing that I would be there for him again, so he would not have to be alone, would help bring a positive attitude. Through no choice of her own, Rachael had to work to pay their bills so was unable to be by his side as much as she wanted to so that she could give the full support he desperately seemed to need.

Considering the physical and emotional turmoil he had been through I was amazed to hear him so upbeat and happy. I was thankful and tried to keep the same upbeat attitude. I wondered in the back of my mind if he was also holding back from showing any negative emotions so he would also appear to be the strong one. Or was it that he was just so happy to be alive and standing there that day?

Chapter 6
September 2001

We Will Be There

Sometimes life hands out the worst
It seems you will never cope
Feeling inside that you are going to burst
Where is that last ray of hope

When life hands out that bitterness
And you want to cry "help" out loud
Do not give in to sadness
There is a hand reaching out in the crowd

That hand is reaching out to you
It will meet you half the way
It cannot tell you what to do
But will be there each and every day

Just to hug and hold and help out
Someone to tell your troubles to
There is no question, without a doubt
You know we will do all we can do

I will say a prayer for you at night
And stand right by your side
To help relieve sadness and fright
Your family we are with pride

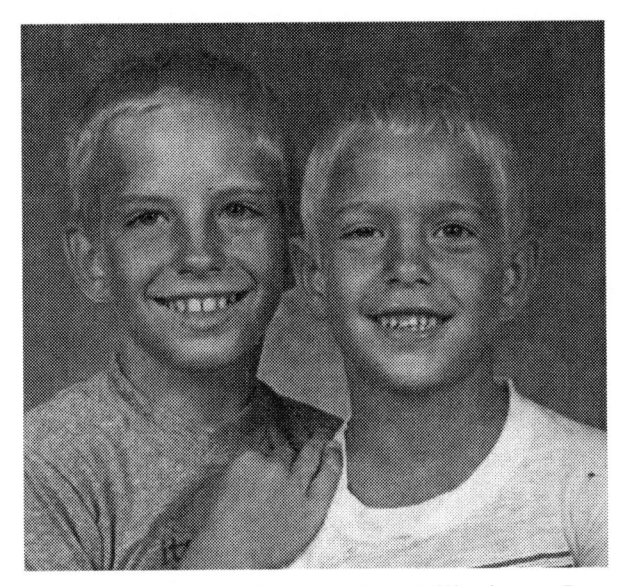

Best Friends and Brothers We Will Always Be

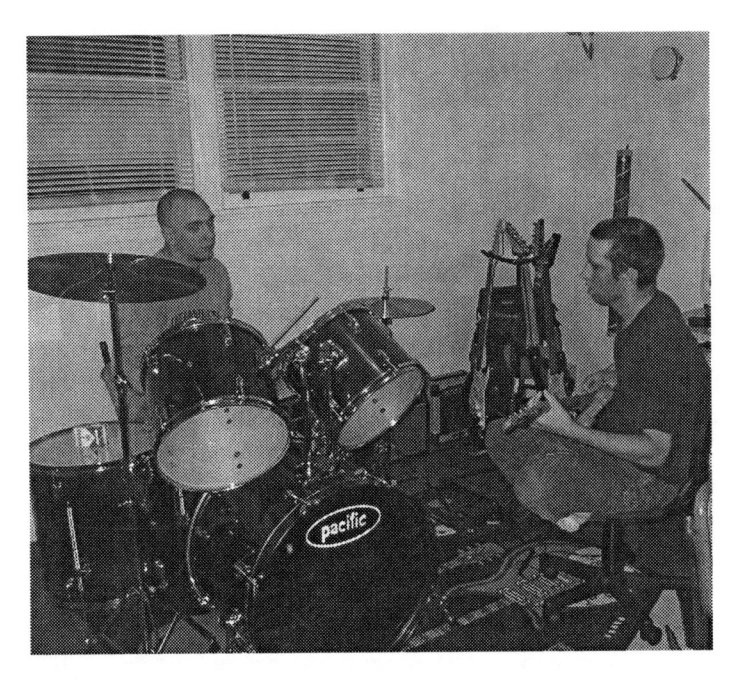

A Favorite Pastime Shared Together

The following day I drove Chad to the hospital for admission for round three of chemotherapy. We were welcomed with open arms from the wonderful nursing staff. The nurses were becoming more like family to us as time passed by. They were understanding but yet kept their emotional distance. I understood this, as I had been an oncology nurse in the past. I, like them, had been told to not get emotionally involved with the patients and their families.

There were two very special nurses that requested taking care of Chad whenever they were on duty. Chad had taken a liking to Elizabeth as he could play his antics on her and she would see the humor in it. She also became someone special that he could talk to in confidence and trust. Their personalities played off each other in a unique way. The other was Amy. Amy had become my "hospital daughter." She and Chad talked as a brother and sister would. She cared not only for Chad but for any needs that I might have that she could help with. All the nursing staff on the fifth floor was wonderful but these two seemed to be able to meet Chad's medical and emotional needs the best. They could help keep him in a positive outlook towards his recovery. Over time we came to know Elizabeth and Amy well enough that there is no way they could not get emotionally involved with our family and us with them.

Chad was shown to his room where he once again "modeled" his white hospital gown with the little blue designs. First came the miles of paperwork that had to be done with each and every admission. Chad and I talked often of how they had everything already there but still he had to go through the same routine for admission every time. All the lab work was completed and the IV's started.

Soon the nausea and vomiting started in once again rearing its ugly head. Different medications for nausea, vomiting and pain were tried to see if they could find the right combination of drugs that would work to keep Chad as comfortable as possible. He preferred anything that would help him to just sleep through it. I had no problem with that if it would help him handle the situation and side effects from the chemotherapy.

When Chad was trying to rest I would spend time reading, writing, watching television or occasionally getting a nap in for myself. At times I would let the nursing staff know I was going out to get outside of the four walls to walk around the hospital grounds. I felt guilty getting to be outside but needed the break to keep my sanity to be strong for Chad. I left my cell phone number with the nursing staff so if I was needed while walking out on

HOLDING ON FOR DEAR LIFE

the hospital grounds or at the cafeteria/snack bar. They never needed to call but then I was never gone for more than fifteen to twenty minutes at a time.

Neither Chad nor I had much contact with the outside world except by telephone. Our cellular phones became our lifeline to family and friends. At the time of Chad's onset of his illness I just had local service on my cellular phone. Upon receiving my monthly bill from the first chemotherapy stay in Atlanta I went into a new anxiety attack. The bill was over four hundred dollars. I stood outside the hospital and contacted my cellular phone carrier. I explained the situation to them and by the grace of God they offered to cut the bill in half. With their help and suggesting I also set up my service to include long distance calls. I knew God was going to take care of my needs while I cared for His child for sure now. If I were to lose my lifeline to family and friends I would have had a much more difficult emotional time.

Rachael would come up to the hospital to be with Chad after her day's work on most evenings. The three of us would sit and watch television together and visit or I would leave the room for awhile so that the two of them could have some time alone. There were not a lot of places to go to in the hospital in the evening hours but I found a few.

I had no question in my mind that the two of them were meant to be a couple. Through her fear of the situation Rachael could have walked away from this but chose to stand by Chad's side. Her love for him was strong. Her strength and faith were strong. Chad's love for Rachael was just as strong. They were definitely soul mates put together in union by God.

Our hospital stay for the chemotherapy this time was just short of a week. Chad was released after the chemotherapy and we returned to their apartment to start taking his temperature every four hours so that we would know if and when to go to the hospital.

Five days later he and I were rushing through the streets of Atlanta in the early morning hours to get to the emergency room. Once again a fever overtook him with signs of infection. After paperwork was complete and examination done, Chad was taken up to his assigned room on the fifth floor.

As soon as Chad was gowned and settled in his hospital bed the nurse came in and started an IV antibiotic. He seemed to be resting easily. After the adrenaline rush I had had it was difficult for me to sleep right away. With each trip to the hospital the fear of him dying before we got there grew stronger. Two hours passed and Chad began to complain about being short of breath. I rang the buzzer for the nurse.

"I can't breathe, Mom," were Chad's next gasping words. "I can't wait for the nurse; go get her."

I ran to the nurses' station and brought the nurse back to the room quickly. She did a quick assessment of the situation and stopped the IV antibiotic and placed him on oxygen. It was an allergic reaction. Chad was monitored often and after a few hours longer was breathing normally again and seemed to be resting well with his eyes closed.

I had prayed almost constantly through that night but had one more to say before I finally laid my weary body down onto the chair bed to get some sleep with seeing the dawn's early light. It started out with "Thank you, God, for letting me keep my son…"

The days once again passed by slowly. By now the nursing staff was starting to discover which combinations of medications were helpful to Chad in controlling his pain, nausea and vomiting. He was now starting to have longer times between the vomiting and seemed to be resting better when he did sleep.

Daily the lab team came in and drew blood from him and we watched and waited for his blood counts to go up. IV fluids continued and the standard for his recovery was to give him bags of blood and/or platelets at least every third day while in the hospital. Receiving all this blood and platelets was of some concern with allergic reactions, AIDS and other illnesses. Overall this was a minimal concern compared to the other problems he was facing. Once again there was really no choice; it seemed that every decision we were given to make was a matter of hoping the treatment would help him to live or let him die. And sadly the alternative with either decision could cause him to die. By now his body was feeling the effects of all the chemotherapy and he was becoming very weak.

My breaks from hospital life came on Friday or Saturday evenings depending on Rachael's work schedule. Rachael would bring a home-cooked meal for us. We were encouraged to get Chad to eat anything we could or that he wanted as his appetite had all but diminished. After eating I would depart with difficulty, even though I knew the break was needed and Chad would be well watched over by Rachael. It was just the fear of something going wrong, like him dying, and me not being by his side. I knew my fear was real because it would only take from one minute to the next for something to go wrong. I knew that Chad also welcomed the break and looked forward to him and Rachael spending time alone.

Driving down the streets of Atlanta in the dark made me miss not having a support person by my side. Emotions seem to be higher and stronger when you are alone and it is the darkness of night. Once at the apartment I really felt very alone. My other problems of finances and my relationship with my fiancé would surface. At least when I was at the hospital I could put them on a back burner and concentrate on Chad. Rachael and I did not get to spend much time together. We would be like passing ships in the night.

Chad and Rachael's Boston terrier, Mattie, and her three cats were my welcoming committee and would greet me at the apartment door on my arrival. In some small way they were a comfort. I then would shower, do laundry and repack for the next week ahead before retiring to the darkness of the night. It felt good to sleep in a bed and stretch out. During the week my bed remained a chair in the corner of Chad's hospital room that folded down. It was far from comfortable and there was no rolling over or stretching out. But at least I was able to stay at his side in his room and get some rest at night. It was not a matter of options in my mind. It was where I belonged and where I wanted to be. How much sleep we got would depend on how Chad's night went and how restless I was feeling with all that my mind was busy with.

On either Saturday or Sunday afternoon I would return to the hospital, once again depending on Rachael's work schedule. Sometimes I would go out and do a little shopping and other times I would just relax at the apartment or the complex pool. It was good for me to get out around society. I never was there long enough to socialize but was good to see people in surroundings outside the hospital area. I was reluctant to get very close to anyone for fear I would then be a carrier for something deadly to Chad. I appreciated being able to be about in society now after seeing how confined Chad had to be living his life. I almost felt anger towards them as I watched people be active and laugh and enjoy being alive. I often wondered if any of them realized how blessed they really were.

All the times away from Chad I still remained on edge for fear of a phone call that Chad may take a turn for the worse, which could happen in just a matter of minutes or seconds. It always felt good to be driving back to the hospital. Chad was always doing okay when I would return as he was in good care with Rachael, but it was comforting to be back by his side.

After two weeks in the hospital and more Neupogen shots to help Chad's body to raise his blood counts, the numbers finally started approaching normal range. Finally they were high enough for Chad to get to go home and he felt better emotionally. The first thing Chad wanted to do was to go get his hair taken care of. By this time he had lost most of his beautiful thick locks of light brown hair. He now only had little stubbles of hair left about his head.

While in the hospital his hair first began coming out in his comb and then he could run his fingers through it and would have a handful. He enjoyed teasing the nurses when they came in, especially the student nurses. He would run his fingers through his hair and show them the handfuls. They would freak out and not knowing what to say or do they would go inform Elizabeth, his nurse they were training under. The nurse along with us would get a good chuckle out of it. In the amusement and seeing how it was entertaining to Chad, Elizabeth did not discourage him.

Chad had a sparkle in his eye as he teased the nursing assistants and nursing students with his magical way of removing his hair. It reminded me of how he loved magic and how it would put a sparkle in his eye to amaze others. One of his most precious memories was when I took him to see a famous magician on stage for his birthday and after the show he got to meet and get a picture taken with him.

That event led to Chad's interest in wanting to learn magic at the early age of seven. We found a magic store in Oklahoma City where, with the assistance of the owner, we purchased several tricks that were appropriate for his age and size of hands. I also found a retired magician that was willing to give Chad lessons. To this day I do not know how he did one of his tricks. "A magician never tells his secrets," Chad would tell me after he started taking lessons. The only secrets to the tricks he let me in on were the ones where he needed my assistance. When his teacher thought he was good enough to go on stage Chad got stage-fright and did not want to take lessons anymore. Often over the years he would still perform his magic for family and friends.

Reality that he was going to lose all his hair really set in when Chad took a shower and the tub was full of hair. Maintenance had to be called because the tub would not drain. Almost all of it was gone except for a few strands on top. This was an emotional time for him. I made a point to collect some of his hair and placed it into an envelope just as I had when he was an infant and gotten his first haircut.

Though it was a hard thing to accept, Chad still found humor in becoming bald without having to pay someone to shave his head. Rachael and I reassured Chad that he had a very nicely shaped head, which he truly did. I reminded him that Shawn was going to shave his head as soon as Chad lost his hair. They could both grow new hair back together. Chad smiled and then laughed. He could not wait to see his brother and look at each other with bald heads.

In speaking with Shawn I found out that one of his friends he worked with knew of what was going on and shaved his head "for the cause." Some of his friends also knew of Shawn's plan and reason and also shaved their heads.

Later I discovered that Jeremy and the men he worked with all shaved their heads "for the cause" also. What an awesome way of showing how much they cared and were supporting him.

Chad voiced how he wished he could carve a pumpkin when he got home since Halloween was only a few weeks away now. Before we departed the hospital Rachael purchased a pumpkin for us to make a jack-o-lantern for him. Chad was still not able to be around any fresh fruits or vegetables due to his counts being low. He sat in the living room on the couch and watched from a distance as we carved the pumpkin for him at the dining room table. We spoke of past Halloweens and how one year it was cold and snowy in Kansas and I bundled the boys up for trick or treating. The boys adorned their costumes even though they would be completely covered with winter outerwear. It did not matter to them that you could not see their costumes as long as they did not have to miss out on the free candy. Carving the pumpkin was something that Chad always enjoyed doing as he would cut out a very intricate picture on the pumpkin. The only thing he did not like was placing his hand inside to clean the "goo" out of the center.

Once the pumpkin was completed and given the "Chad seal of approval," Rachael placed it outside the front door as I prepared the seeds for roasting and bagged the remains to be taken directly out to the garbage.

It was now time for me to prepare for my return back to Kansas once again. Back to work and to be with Shawn and my fiancé until the next call would be received.

The morning I was to depart to go back to Kansas we were watching the morning news. A man had darted past the security checkpoint at the Atlanta airport and would not stop when they yelled at him. Due to heightened security since the 9/11 incident the airport was shut down. Everyone inside was evacuated to the outside and the roads to the airport blocked off. I called the airlines to let them know that I could not even get close to the airport due to roads in and out being shut down. They courteously changed my ticket for my flight to the next morning at no charge to myself and thanked me for my call as they had not yet been informed of the airport incident.

The following morning I departed and was back in Kansas to see what the situation had developed into there since I had been gone. I had not been able to reach my fiancé' so I called him periodically to leave a message on the answering machine to let him know what was going on. Now that things were settling down for Chad until his next treatment I needed to get other things settled down in my life.

Chapter 7
November 2001

Where Are You

My son, where are you coming from
Is it someplace where others can come
Is it far away from here
Sometimes it seems you are very near

In your eyes I see for miles
Going further with each tear it cries
The silence of the distant drum
Sometimes it makes you feel so numb

That empty room you have inside
A place where sometimes you run and hide
Continually you are searching to get out
As others think you are sitting to pout

That hurt inside you begs for a cure
To make your heavy heart so pure
To just end it all would be all wrong
So what do you do when it hurts all day long

There is nothing we two cannot overcome
That is what He said; the Bible from
Take one step forward on each day
Let Him carry you the rest of the way

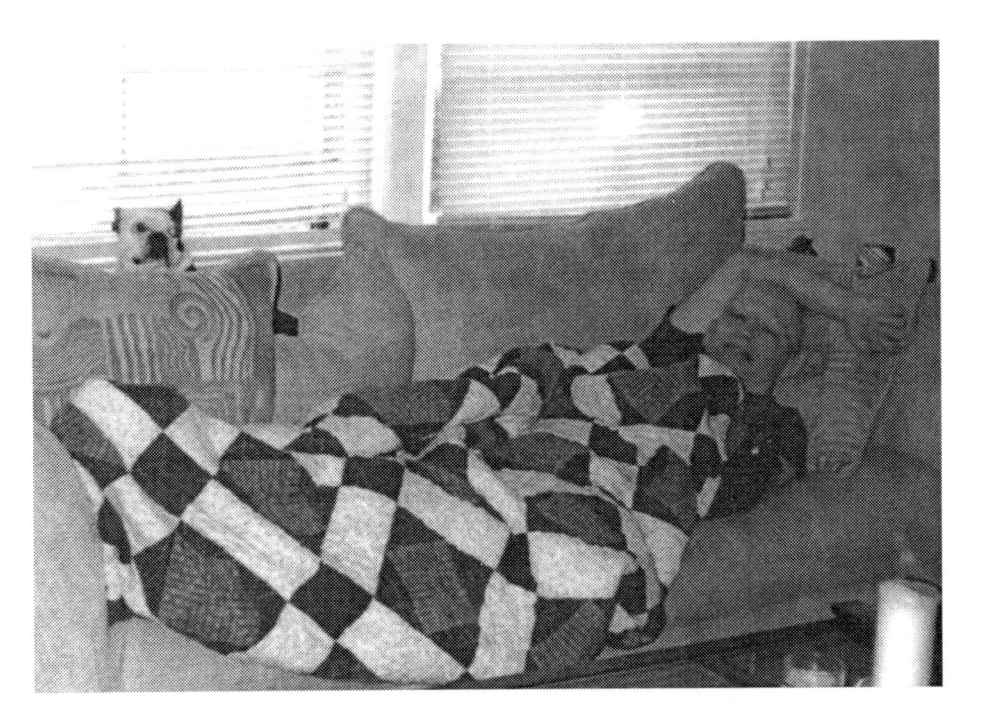

Chad Very Ill and Still Smiling as Mattie Keeps by His Side

While I was back in Kansas, Chad informed me that they were going to be moving from the apartment to a house north of Atlanta. He and Rachael were excited to tell me that they had found a house that would have a mom's room. Chad voiced his concerns of attempting to make the move. He had little strength and the fear of a cut or bruise was very real. He was still weak and on the blood thinner medication.

I had been listening frequently to a Christian radio station in Atlanta so I contacted the manager. In speaking with him and discussing the situation he felt they perhaps could be of some help. To my delight they announced the need for help and Chad received several phone calls from people willing to help with the move. The move was completed without much difficulty and in a very short time. Most importantly, with no damage done to the most precious cargo of the move, Chad.

We kept in touch often and soon I received the call to book another flight. Returning to Atlanta for Chad's next round of chemotherapy brought on a new challenge. I would have to learn how to get from the middle of the city to the north end and find their new home. It was a challenge I was not looking forward to. If you have ever driven in Atlanta you know exactly what I am talking about. I had finally mastered the drive from the hospital to their apartment and now it would be a new challenge with new directions.

Upon arriving into Atlanta Chad and Rachael took me to a furniture store because they wanted me to help select the new mattress set for in "Mom's room." I was pleased that Rachael would welcome me into her and Chad's world with love and open arms. I then went shopping to get a dresser and mirror for in the room.

Once again Chad and I made our drive to the hospital for his admission. This time the chemotherapy seemed to go much easier for Chad. He still had nausea and vomiting but he was kept fairly sedated to ease through it all a little easier. The nursing staff had finally found the combination of medications to keep him as comfortable as could be expected.

By now we were starting to see a pattern. About one to two weeks out from chemotherapy we could plan to have a bag packed for a night trip to the emergency room for admission. Once Chad's immune system was gone he would start running a high fever. Speeding through the middle of Atlanta, Georgia, down highway 75 was not too difficult in the late night or very early morning hours. Only semi trucks seemed to own the road at that time of night.

My heart raced as fast as the engine of Chad's car as I constantly prayed and glanced over at Chad while keeping eyes on the road and ears open for any changes or unusual noises that he might make. It never seemed to get any easier to make those night drives. I was well aware of how quickly an infection could take over his body if not treated immediately since he had no defenses.

We arrived at the emergency room around eleven-thirty. In the emergency room we were seated a little distance from the other waiting patients due to Chad's condition. It was difficult for me to understand why they would have him "wait his turn" when he was so ill and the risks involved. The doctor's words rang in my ears echoing, "We lose more patients from infections while they are neutropenic than we do from the cancer itself."

At last a nurse came to get us. We were directed to an exam room where Chad was placed on a gurney bed. No comfort for him there. A blanket was placed on him for warmth.

After several minutes someone came in to get his vital signs (temperature, pulse and blood pressure) and to tell us a doctor would be in to see him soon. After many more minutes that seemed like hours the emergency room doctor came in to see Chad. The doctor ordered for blood work to be done. Then the doctor told us we would have to wait until the infectious disease specialist came in to see Chad next before he could go up to a room. I did not understand why he could not see Chad in a room on the fifth floor.

After another long wait the infectious disease specialist finally arrived to see Chad. By this time it was around two in the morning. Once he completed his examination he gave orders to the nurse to have blood cultures drawn and then for him to be admitted to the cancer ward, words we were glad to hear. Finally we were going to be able to get him treatment and some rest. We were both extremely tired as it was now almost four o'clock in the morning by this time.

After another wait the nurse announced that the room was ready. An emergency room assistant came with a wheelchair to take Chad to his room. She stopped the wheelchair in front of the nurses' station to get the paperwork that was to go with Chad to his room. The nurse requested a final set of vital signs before departure.

Chad sat partially slumped with a blanket around his shoulders and another over his legs. He was looking so tired and pale by this time. He had not gotten any rest and the infection was increasingly taking over his body. Then he spoke words that sent extreme fear through my entire body.

"Mom, I feel funny," Chad said softly to me, as he seemed to be laboring for his breath and slumped over more in the chair. "My heart feels like it is racing and I can't get my breath."

The assistant immediately wheeled Chad into an empty exam room across from the nurse's station to get his vital signs. She held Chad's wrist for a few seconds then stepped over to the nurse. I heard her tell the nurse that the heartbeat was too fast for her to count. The nurse instructed her to try again and also to get his blood pressure.

By now fear was generating though my entire body as I watched the electronic device monitor the vital signs. My body was shaking and I felt like I was chilling. The blood pressure was one hundred seven over thirty-six, the heart rate was one hundred sixty and respirations were eighteen. I knew this was a sign of distress of some kind. The assistant spoke loudly to the nurse who came quickly and rushed Chad back to the exam room he had just been removed from. At once there were four emergency personnel at his bedside. He was placed quickly back onto the gurney and an EKG connected to him for the reading of his heart beats and rhythm.

Tears welled in my eyes and my heart raced and pounded hard in my chest as I stood just outside the door of the exam room and saw them place his frail pale body onto the gurney. He was reconnected to the electrical device that would monitor his vital signs and check for oxygen rate. Oxygen was placed on his nose through a tube. I began to pray. I prayed hard.

"God, please don't take my son away from me. Not now after he has been through so much to get this far."

I opened my eyes to see the nurse giving Chad some pills of some sort. Something was said about potassium and electrolytes but I could not make out everything as they had me standing too far back outside the room so that I would not be in the way. I knew that if I stayed in the room I would have been in their way anyway because the exam rooms were small.

I felt nausea overtake my stomach and a severe headache rushed through my head. The old expression of "having the crap scared out of you" became a reality. I quickly spotted the restroom sign and ran to the door. Yes, I made it in time. Again I prayed for Chad. The thought went through my mind of if I had to call Rachael and Shawn and tell her he had not survived. Tears flowed down my cheeks.

Upon returning to the emergency room hall beside the exam room I could see that Chad seemed to be resting better. His breathing seemed much less labored. He still had the oxygen tubing in his nose but the EKG machine had been removed. I stepped to his side and kissed him on the forehead.

"How are you feeling now?" I asked.

"Better," was his reply with a soft weak voice. "I just want to get to my room."

In just a few minutes Chad was placed on a stretcher and transported to his room on the fifth floor cancer ward.

We felt relieved to be back on the fifth floor with familiar faces that knew Chad and his care needs. Chad was settled into his bed, an IV was started and more blood draws were done. At this point I began to relax and prepare the room with our belongings knowing it was going to be a long stay again. By now Chad was beginning to feel some better and relaxing more also. I felt we were through with the scare and all was going to be better now. Chad was resting as well as could be expected with all he had been through. We were both becoming more at ease knowing how his body would react and what to expect. Yet I constantly stayed on guard for anything new that might develop. This was all new territory for us and surprises were not usually pleasant anymore.

I felt I was handling as much emotion and stress as I thought my body and mind could handle by now. Little did I know that more was to come with one phone call I made later that evening. Rachael was with Chad in his room and I wanted to give them some "alone" time. I went out to the pay phone in the waiting area to call my fiancé.

I was attempting to tell him of the events that were going on with Chad. I could not believe what my ears were hearing. He was talking of breaking our engagement.

I became hurt and angry on top of all the other feelings I was having. At some point during the conversation I decided that I had enough stress to take care of without worrying about this too. Perhaps it was because I was so tired or that my body and mind could not handle any more than it already was. I would approach this subject in a few weeks when I returned to Kansas. Chad was the number one priority and that was my purpose for being there. His life was more important than my own personal relationship right now.

During one of my daily walks outside the hospital I met a lady whose husband had been admitted to the hospital the previous day that was diagnosed also with cancer. It was a different kind of cancer than Chad had but it was still deadly. We talked extensively for short periods of time each day. When one of us was ready and in need of a walk or talk we would call the other's hospital room and meet outside. It was good to have someone to talk to that was going through the same kinds of emotions that I was.

After our three-week hospital stay Chad was once again released to return home. His counts were coming back up and he was getting over his infection. To monitor him closely he had to go get lab work done and receive blood or platelets daily for four days as an outpatient. Our daily morning trips to the blood center at the hospital were still much better for Chad than staying within the four walls of a hospital room. His outlook improved the moment he would arrive inside his home.

I contacted Shawn and set up plans for him and his girlfriend to fly out to Atlanta so that we could be together as a family for Shawn's birthday, Christmas and New Years. It would be the first time the boys had seen each other since this all started in June.

Chad expressed his excitement of having Shawn there with him. It was a good boost to Chad's outlook to have the support of his brother by his side. One of their special things was for one of them to ask, "Where do they go?" and the other to say "Silo." It was a running joke between the two of them like several others that they had. The closeness and love between the two brothers was unsurpassed.

I purchased plane tickets for Shawn and his girlfriend, Cathy, to arrive in Atlanta the day before Christmas. I was excited to have my little family back together again.

Christmas morning was a wonderful time although Chad looked back on it and could not remember any of the details. We all gathered in the living room to open gifts. Even though they were few, each gift was special.

One of the effects of the chemotherapy treatments seemed to be loss of memory and lapses in recall, another side effect we had not been made aware of until after the fact.

One evening we all went shopping at a toy store so Shawn could try and find some sea monkeys. While we were there Chad and Shawn played with several of the toys making us all laugh. Chad always seemed to be the instigator. He was not afraid of embarrassing himself or anyone else if it was all in fun. After our little shopping spree we then all went out to eat seafood to celebrate Shawn's birthday. He was turning the big nineteen. It was wonderful to see Chad living life at his fullest again. It was wonderful to see my two sons enjoying each other's company so much. They were talking and scheming and planning and joking with each other just like they had before any of this nightmare had started. I felt blessed having my little family all together again. Chad was once again laughing and joking around keeping smiles on all our faces.

New Year's Eve night found Rachael and me in bed sleeping but Shawn, Cathy and Chad remained up to share the moment of seeing another year arrive. I had purchased some non-alcoholic champagne so that we could celebrate and include Chad. A mistake made and noted; it was inexpensive and it tasted terrible.

All too soon it was January 2002 and time for Shawn and Cathy to return to Kansas. I would be following behind them at the end of the week after Chad's next doctor visit.

With the completion of another round of chemotherapy for Chad and getting past being neutropenic, it was time for me to board a plane and return to Kansas once again. I made a call to Valerie to let her know when the plane I was on would be arriving so that she could pick me up at the airport.

I was surprised that the airlines employees were not calling me by my first name on approach to the ticket counter by now. The two-hour flight was okay but I always dreaded the five-hour drive back to my hometown once I landed at the airport in Kansas City. The drive seemed even longer this time because I had relationship problems that would have to be addressed. Up until now I had not given it much thought, as I was too busy tending to the business at hand of helping Chad to live. I was tired and emotionally exhausted and now I would have to deal with finding out what was going on with my relationship with my fiancé. But before driving back home Valerie prepared a meal for us and a bed for me to sleep in for a good night's rest. It was always heartwarming to return back to the comforting words and kindness of family.

Chapter 8
January 2002

I Found a Friend

I thought life would always be my friend
Right up to the very end
Through thick and thin every day
Always giving me a tomorrow on the way

The years passed quickly; as they do
Now in time of need I call on you
I thought you would help me out
That I could depend on you without a doubt

I reached out, you slapped my hand
I needed a rock, you gave me sand
I needed a hug, away you ran
I needed you to reassure that "I can"

You taught me a lesson I thank you for
If you're in trouble life may slam a door
In my search I found a door to knock
It opened and I was given a rock

I reached out, He squeezed my hand
I needed a hug, to me He ran
I needed a song, He sent me a band
I needed reassurance, He said "You can"

HOLDING ON FOR DEAR LIFE

I received the faith and strength I needed
The grains of love and understanding He seeded
He said He would always be my faithful friend
Even AFTER the very end

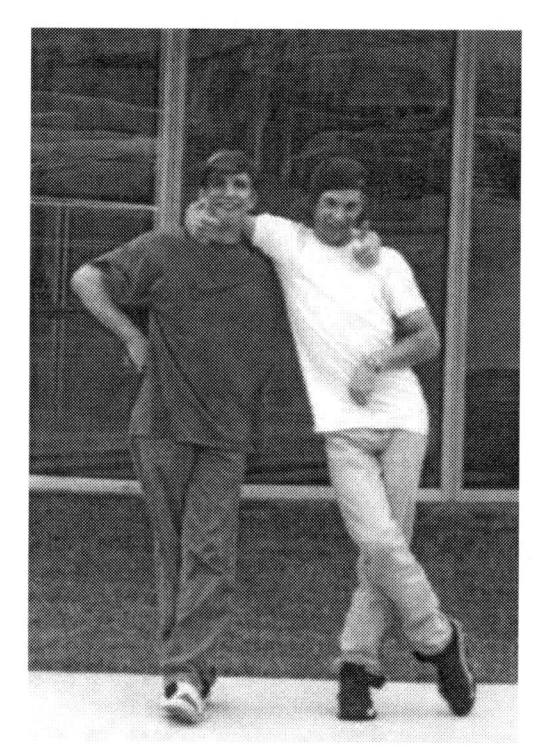

Brotherly Love, Fun and Bonding

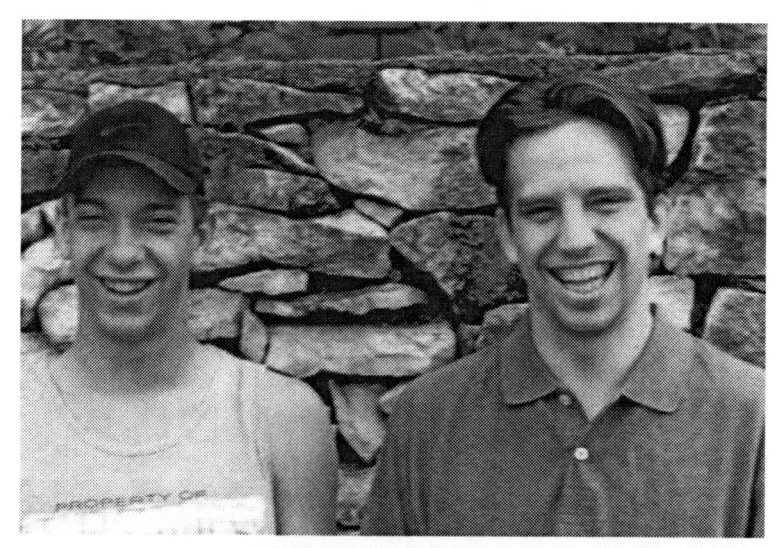

Best of Friends Beyond the End

I was not sure what kind of reception I would receive on returning to the house. My fiancé and I had been living together for almost three years and now a decision would have to be made as to if it was truly over or if we could work through this. As I walked up to the front door of the house I took a deep breath. I opened the door and entered in. I expected him to be waiting for me but there was no one home.

Strangely it was relaxing to me to be alone in quietness. As I was unpacking my bags I heard the front storm door open. I stood still listening and waiting but no one entered the bedroom where I was. No one called out to me. "It is over," I said to myself. I had been home only a short time when Shawn came over to welcome me back.

I began a search to get my own place for a little while for us to see if we could get our lives back in order. We agreed that we would stay engaged and date to see if that would bring the relationship back to where it once was.

I proceeded to find a two-bedroom place and asked Shawn to move in with me. He had pretty much been on his own over the past year and even more so after he had returned to Kansas with his aunt Tina, when Chad was first diagnosed. He had moved into an apartment with a friend of his when he returned. It was wonderful to have him close to me again. We had a chance to make up for lost times spent doing things together as mother and son. I do not doubt that he felt pretty deserted since I was a single parent and he had to abruptly fend for himself at age eighteen. There were family members he could contact there in town if needed but was always one to try and do for himself. Shawn had new adventures and learned experiences to share with me on each of my return visits. He had questions for me regarding his search for answers to some of life's dilemmas. It was a joy having this time to share life with him again.

The dividing of the house with my fiancé and me increased the end of the relationship. I felt relief in my own place to not feel like I was under fire or stressed and graciously accepted my time for myself.

I called Georgia regularly while back in Kansas to make sure all was going well. I would get reports of new hair growth, increased appetite and activity and weight gain. Reports of new restaurants they tried, a trip to the mall to window shop or a new movie they went to see was always good to hear. It appeared that everything was normal, as if nothing had ever happened.

But then all too soon again I received the phone call of when the next chemotherapy treatment would be started. I had my routine down by now. Pack my suitcase, call the airlines, make arrangements for transportation to the airport, and call family members and my boss to let them know of the schedule.

My heart felt a little lighter as I boarded the plane to take me to Atlanta this time. I felt positive that we were home free after this last round of chemotherapy and being neutropenic. It also helped that we had learned from the previous treatments how to handle the situations easier. It did not help keep the anxiety or fear away but we did understand better of what was going on. It seemed we had managed to survive the worst-case scenario.

As I approached baggage claim in the Atlanta airport I saw Chad and Rachael waiting for me. There was a smile on Chad's face and he was his cheerful self. The grin on his face was one I had not seen in a long time. It was the look of knowing something special that he could not wait to share with me. I had seen that look on his face many times as a child. As I got closer Chad lifted off his baseball cap to show me that he once again had a full head of hair. Though not very long, it was all over his head. He was so proud.

Since Chad was between the time of being neutropenic and having chemotherapy he could get out into society as long as it was not around a large crowd of people. We went to the computer store so that Chad could get himself a laptop computer. This would give him more connections with the outside world that he so desperately needed while he was in the hospital. It was good for him to have contact with his friends and family. That would re-enforce that others cared and were praying for him, even if they could not be there with him.

During treatments Chad sometimes felt that no one really cared about him since he did not receive many phone calls and had had no visits from any other family members or friends. He did understand the problems of making trips with consideration to time, distance and money but it did not seem to ease his feeling of being forgotten sometimes. At times I would remind him of someone calling to talk to him that his recall memory did not recall. Much of this seemed to stem from the depression that would overtake him with each hospital admission.

Chad sensed my feelings of loneliness at times also. He suggested to me that I get on the internet and find friends to talk with that way. I was reluctant because I had heard many stories of bad happenings from contacts with people one might meet on the internet. He persistently reassured me that it would be fine and showed me how to get on to locate people to talk with. He also gave me a verbal list of his internet rules for chatting safely.

I did find someone to talk to that was a kind, religious person that lived a little over two hours from Atlanta. After Chad was in bed for the night I would get on the computer and talk with my newfound friend. His name was Monty. Monty was understanding and patient. Our talks helped me to keep my mind and feelings in check when I thought I was going to fall apart or became upset about something. After six months of occasional chatting on the computer we finally started talking over the phone. Over the course of time Monty became a very good friend.

Rarely, but on occasion it does snow in the south. We awoke one morning to hear on the news that snow was expected. As afternoon approached the snow did begin to fall. We watched the news reports that flashed across the television as if a tornado was approaching. The total snowfall was about two inches. The entire city of Atlanta pretty much shut down. All television channels kept everyone posted all day of closings, road conditions, etc. This seemed odd to us as we came from the Midwest where even a foot of snow would not keep you from work most of the time.

As I was watching the snow fall out the window I thought back to the day Chad was born. On the morning of February 25, 1977, in Oklahoma I gave birth to a beautiful baby boy. By that afternoon we had a large amount of snow fall as the wind blew the large flakes around. I recalled how I felt warm and cozy as I lay in a hospital bed holding my eight-pound baby boy. He had big blue eyes and dark brown hair. I marveled at his little hands and feet and thanked God that he had ten fingers and toes. He was perfect in every way. I thought a prayer right then and there was needed to thank God for letting me be the one selected to be Chad's mother and prayed for his complete recovery from this horrible trial he was going through.

By the following morning in Atlanta there was not a trace to be seen anywhere to remind anyone of the winter snow that had fallen the day before.

The afternoon before his hospital admission, Chad got another treat. He enjoyed going to the movies and we went to a movie matinee. It was heart warming to see him enjoy the simple things in life that we all take for granted. Walks around the mall and an afternoon movie matinee were a treat and exciting for him now. The little things we take for granted need to be realized by us that are healthy. We must all learn to cherish even the moments of the simple things and look for the beauty in all things.

Chapter 9

A Light Does Shine

A light shines in the darkness
But seems so far away
At times it seems to shine less
But constantly it does stay

At times the light doth flicker
As if it almost goes out
Sometimes slower, sometimes quicker
But stays lit without a doubt

At times the light shines brightly
Other times it appears so dim
When it shines so ever slightly
I send prayers straight up to Him

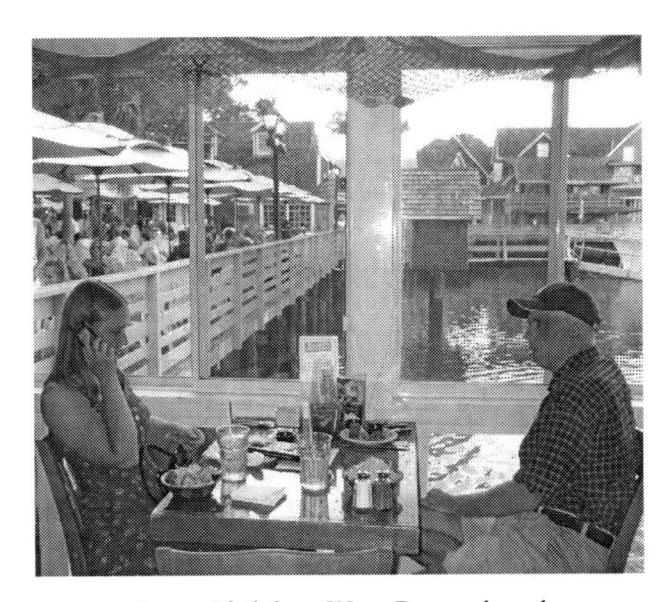

Some Birthdays Were Remembered

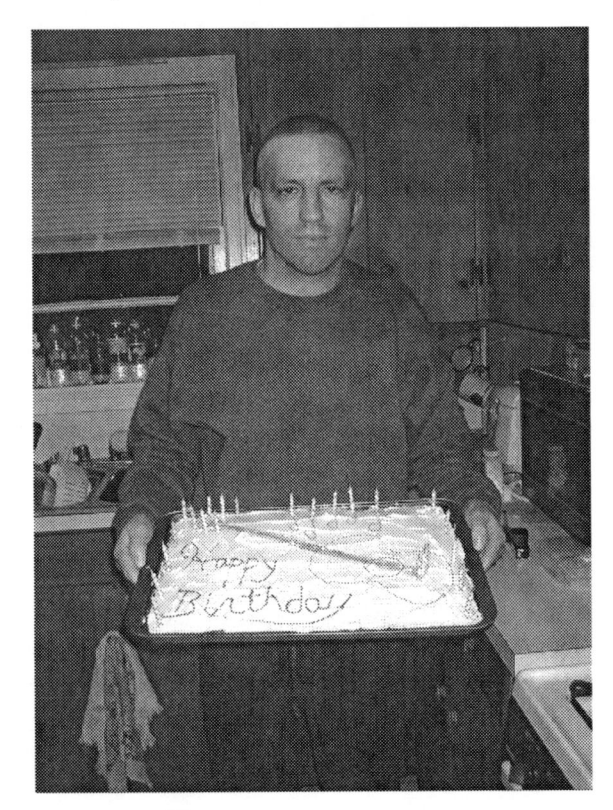

Some Birthdays Were Not

Once again, for what I was hoping was the last time, I took Chad to the hospital for admission for his last round of chemotherapy. Upon admission he was taken to his room where vital signs were taken, lab work done and an IV started for fluids. Often I wondered how much blood they could pull out of him and still leave enough for him to function. Blood draws were a daily routine of at least three vials. An IV was then started with the chemotherapy.

All was going by what was now routine. The nursing staff knew exactly what combination of medications to give him by now to help control the pain and nausea and vomiting.

Chad rested well during the first two days of his chemotherapy induction stay this time. I only wished they could have found that special combination of medication for Chad about four chemotherapy treatments ago. It was a relief to know that Chad was facing his last round of chemotherapy. Chad looked forward to all our lives getting back to normal, as did Rachael and I. He talked of getting to go back to work and doing the normal things he used to do.

With the passing of each episode of chemotherapy the possibility for a wedding was starting to become a reality again. The two of them would now be able to continue their plans for a wedding. Chad had agreed that since he was in remission there was little doubt he would be leaving Rachael a widow as he had feared. His depression was lifting and his outlook was becoming more positive.

The wedding date was now set for June 1, 2002. During this time in the hospital I cheerfully worked on making the ring pillow, flower basket, helped make rice bags and got to go with Rachael as she selected a wedding dress. It was wonderful to get to experience the joys as a fill-in mother of the bride and be the mother of the groom.

I was finally going to get a daughter that I had always wished I had had to fit into the family along with my sons. I was so proud of Chad that he had selected such a wonderful person to join our family. Joy was now replacing some of our fear. Tears of happiness were replacing tears of a broken heart. We were preparing for a day that nine months ago we thought would never happen. I would be blessed with getting the daughter I had always wanted and getting to keep a son.

As the days passed by Chad started becoming more and more ill and unable to eat. I painfully watched daily as he became weaker and sicker. There was not even a day's break for him from the nausea, vomiting and pain. His skin became pale and his eyes dull. I longed to see that sparkle in his eyes.

The medication regimen did not seem to be helping as it had earlier. His strength had to come from deep inside just to get up out of his bed. My fear increased that he would have to fight more infection in such a weak condition.

Chad's complexion was becoming ashy yet had sort of a yellow tint to it. His skin had become extremely dry and flaky. He had no hair left on his body, not even eyebrows, as he had lost it all again. The sparkle in his eyes was replaced by a dull haze that sometimes carried a blank stare.

My heart ached for him and I frequently fought back tears. I only nodded off on occasion through the day and night as he would become confused and get up to go to the restroom and forget he was in the hospital and was connected to an IV.

This was the last chemotherapy treatment and things were getting worse. He was so close to recovery and yet it was beginning to appear that he may not recover. Numerous lab tests were being done in an attempt to determine the cause of Chad becoming so ill.

My times to cry were alone in the patient family room or outside. I had found a place beside the hospital that had a few seating benches that were mostly concealed by tall hedges. I did not want Chad to see my fear because I was afraid it would show him that I had my doubts of his recovery. I still felt I needed to be the strong one to help him keep a positive attitude. The friend I had met previously that her husband had cancer had left the hospital shortly after Chad's last dismissal. There was no one to share feelings with at the hospital now when I went outside for awhile.

There was no one to sit beside me, so I looked to Heaven. Faith began growing stronger with each prayer that I prayed. I searched for answers but seemed to get few responses to come into my head. That did not keep me from becoming determined that prayers and faith would see this through. It only takes faith the size of a mustard seed to move a mountain, I reminded myself. New hope for Chad's recovery came with each time I prayed.

It became difficult for Chad to eat due to the sores that had developed in his mouth and throat from the chemotherapy. The smell of food made him terribly nauseous. Not until he gave permission was the lid over his food plate even attempted to be lifted when his food tray was brought into his room. Permission was given again that Chad could have anything to eat that he was hungry for. Exceptions were fresh fruits or vegetables that he could not have.

Once again anytime he did become hungry for anything I would leave promptly to go get it in hopes that by the time I did get back with it he would still be hungry for it. On occasions his nausea would return before I could get back to the room and he could not eat anything again. Among his favorites were pizza, chili or chicken fingers. When Rachael would bring home-cooked food for him he would at least give it a good try to eat.

By the third morning of treatment the doctor came in to inform us that Chad's infection was in his blood. There was question of possible cross contamination from another source to his IV port that was in his chest. The word of fear is 'sepses. This was a very serious problem. It meant that his body was trying to fight against a very serious infection. Chad had just gotten his chemotherapy, which meant that his immune system was going to be depleted to zero. His body was not going to have any cells in it to fight this infection that can be deadly to a healthy person.

The doctor had also decided that Chad would have to start getting his nutrition through IV solutions since he was unable to eat. Chad was becoming weaker with each passing day and now starting to lose weight.

After the doctor left the room I waited just a short time and then went out by the nurses' station to find the doctor. I did not want Chad to hear the conversation. I informed the doctor that I was scheduled to fly back to Kansas in two days but because of Chad's condition I was skeptical about leaving. His words cut deep. "Debbi, this is the worst I have seen Chad. I don't recommend that you leave."

After speaking with him I went to the family room and cried my heart out. I wondered if this time he was going to have the strength to be able to fight hard enough to overcome the battle for as ill as he was becoming. Fear consumed my body once again. I wondered if I should call Shawn to come out. I would have given almost anything at that moment to have someone there to hold me as I cried and to listen to my fears. Once again I only had God there to comfort me and pretty sure that he had sent extra angels our way. I was glad that Chad was not aware of just how ill he was.

Once I got my emotions settled down I called the airlines and canceled my flight and called my boss to let him know I would not be returning to work just yet. He said to not worry and just know that prayers were with us. I had thought that I would return home until Chad became neutropenic but this changed my plans abruptly. I prayed about the situation and decided to wait before bringing Shawn out. I called my friend in Oklahoma and he told me that Chad would make it through this. I rested a little easier but not much.

There was little conversation between Chad and anyone during this time. He was too weak and ill to hardly talk. Rest and medication to keep Chad partially sedated from the pain and sickness were now daily on a set schedule.

The nursing staff had once again found just the right combination of medications to help Chad make it through these times.

I have always been an active person. You know the type, cannot sit and watch a movie on television from beginning to end without getting up to do something. Nervous energy I think was what a doctor told me once. Now I sat in silence and would have to be still. I had learned patience and my faith had grown in leaps and bounds. God knew I needed to learn that but this would not be the way I would have chosen.

As Chad began to sleep more with the aid of medication, the days began to get longer. It sometimes seemed that days would never come to an end. Loneliness became an all-too-familiar friend. Yet in my heart and mind I felt it was such a small price to pay for being by my son's bedside and not his gravesite.

There were times I would have given almost anything to have someone there to talk to as Chad slept. It seemed as though contact with family was seldom by now. I had to limit my calls to keep expenses down. I would occasionally get a call from friends and family. I wondered if it was difficult for others to call because no one wanted to face the fact that Chad would perhaps not survive or that they just did not know what to say. I would send out e-mails as Chad's condition would change to keep them informed. However, there were some that kept close contact.

One afternoon my inner silent loneliness was replaced by sheer joy. The phone rang and when I answered it my cousin Tony's voice was on the other end of the phone. It was a call I will never forget; it came at a time when my heart needed it the most. During Tony's busy day he took the time to pick up the phone and call at one of the times when I needed it most emotionally. I think that God must have encouraged him to do so. It had been a very long time since Tony and I had visited and it filled the emptiness of the silent loneliness. We had a wonderful visit and Tony had me laughing, as he seemed to be talented in that area like Chad was. I now knew how Chad felt and what he meant when he just needed the reassurance that family and friends were still thinking of him and that they cared.

By now my nerves were frayed and stress was taking over my mind and body. I was running with lack of sleep. I approached the doctor to inquire of something to help me handle my nerves. He gave me a prescription. My guard of strength was starting to crumble down. My emotional strength was weakening.

Chad seldom complained through all this. When he did complain of anything it was well justified. Often his tear-filled words haunt me of that night, in the dark when I held him as he said, "Mom, I don't want to die." How he was surviving though all this had to be with God's hand. As he lay there so listless I prayed for God to send his angel Michael with his army of angels to stand around the bed and to fight off any evil that the devil may throw Chad's way. He was too tired, sick and weak and needed some help in fighting this battle. His days were long and his nights restless most of the time. Since that night I realize how small we are in such a great big world. I realized how helpless and alone we are by ourselves in this world. Faith and trust in God is a powerful thing and was all I had to hang on to.

You may be wondering why I do not describe more of Chad's feelings and thoughts during these times. It is because he does not recall them. I do not know if it was because of the drugs he was given or his body's mechanism to cope with all that he was going through or a combination of both. Whatever it was, I thank God for it because it made it easier for Chad to deal with everything he was going through. Even for Rachael and myself there are events that are vivid in our mind but it is difficult to put a time frame on them when we recall them. There are also events that we remind each other about that the other had forgotten. I think the mind has a mechanism to help the human body to be able to heal itself. The heartfelt pain and tears return with each event I must remember and emotion I must relive to write Chad's story.

It took several weeks for Chad to improve. This was a very serious infection he was fighting this time and improvement was slow. At long last he was coming to active life again. The IV nutrition was stopped as his eating began to improve. He was still weak but his strength was increasing slowly over time. We started taking short walks in the hallway and talked more since he was staying awake and alert for longer periods of time. Even when awake Chad did not feel like doing anything active yet that would take much strength. Occasionally, for short periods of time, he would watch a movie, watch television, or get on the Internet to email friends and family or just talk. As Chad's health began to improve he became bored and restless. He desperately wanted to go home.

Two weeks after the chemotherapy treatment was completed Chad got another infection while neutropenic. This time it was the after-chemo infection per schedule. Chad was starting to ask the doctor daily if he could go home. Upon my agreement the doctor said he would release Chad to go home as long as I would administer IV antibiotics to him that he would order. Chad looked at me with hope and desperation in his eyes and I agreed.

I was instructed on the procedure for administering Chad's medications and IV therapy at home. On the same day we arrived to the house the medications, supplies and equipment were delivered to the door. There were several boxes of all sizes. I wondered what I had gotten myself into. The items and equipment were things needed for the IV medications to be administered, medication to flush his port in his chest, IV bags of antibiotic solution that had to be refrigerated and an emergency box. That box was of most concern to me. The home care nurse would be arriving the next morning to instruct me in administering the medications and use of items in the emergency box.

I used every precaution possible in administering the medications. I did not want to take a chance of Chad facing any more infection than he had already had. The thought of me infecting him would put me into an asylum for sure. With each time I administered the medication, Chad would give me words of encouragement that I was doing fine. I was relieved when the last IV bag had finished and the equipment was taken away.

When Chad's blood levels finally returned to normal he was his cheerful fun-loving self again. His personality is one to be treasured. He could make a person laugh and see the humor in almost anything. I still think he would have been magnificent on stage or in movies. Yet there was some personality change since all this began. His temper became short and he could be harsh almost to cruelty with words at times. The medications were taking a new side effect now. There were now times that Chad had no recollection of what happened in his life during certain current events.

In February Chad's birthday came and went. I had made him a cake and we had ice cream. Several months later Chad commented that we had not done anything for his birthday. I got out the pictures I had taken of him with his cake to show him we had celebrated. He stated that it was a good thing I took the pictures because he did not remember any of it. At different times during chemotherapy it was not unusual for Chad's mind to even totally block things out. Nothing I read about leukemia and its treatments said anything about something like this ever happening or how to deal with it.

With the chemotherapy regimen behind Chad and he in remission it was time to return to Kansas. Chad, Rachael and myself were all three ready to put this past behind us and return to normal life routines. Chad would soon be returning to work and Rachael would continue with wedding preparations. Myself, I was glad to return back to a life that I once complained of being boring. Once back in Kansas I called often to make sure all was going well in Georgia, almost to the point of overkill. When Chad and Rachael's phone rang they would look at each other and say, "It's Mom." It was heart lifting for me to hear them tell of times spent out and about. Chad continued to reassure me that he was doing fine. In just three months we would be together again for the wedding.

Worries and fear were finally diminished one month later when another bone marrow biopsy was done to confirm that he was still in remission. There was much to celebrate now as Chad was cancer free and a wedding was soon to take place.

Chapter 10
April 2002

A Wonderful Way to Live

Life is not easy, who said it was
You will hit bottom as everyone does
Start at the bottom to get to the top
Pick yourself up whenever you drop
You have to get up to start each day
And every day has a price you have to pay
You open a door, it slams in your face
People will want to put you "in your place"
Like a diamond that starts rugged and rough
It has to be cut and polished to shine enough
Everything has to struggle to keep alive
You too have to fight to survive
You say this is hard for you to do
You search for an answer, if you only knew
There is someone waiting to help you
To make life easier to live through
You do not have to search, she is right there
She loves you and really does care
Her name is Rachael and you can guess
A true soul mate, no more, no less
She will help take the worry, fear and loneliness
And make it joy, love and peacefulness
Your walk through life will be together
She will be by your side through all kinds of weather

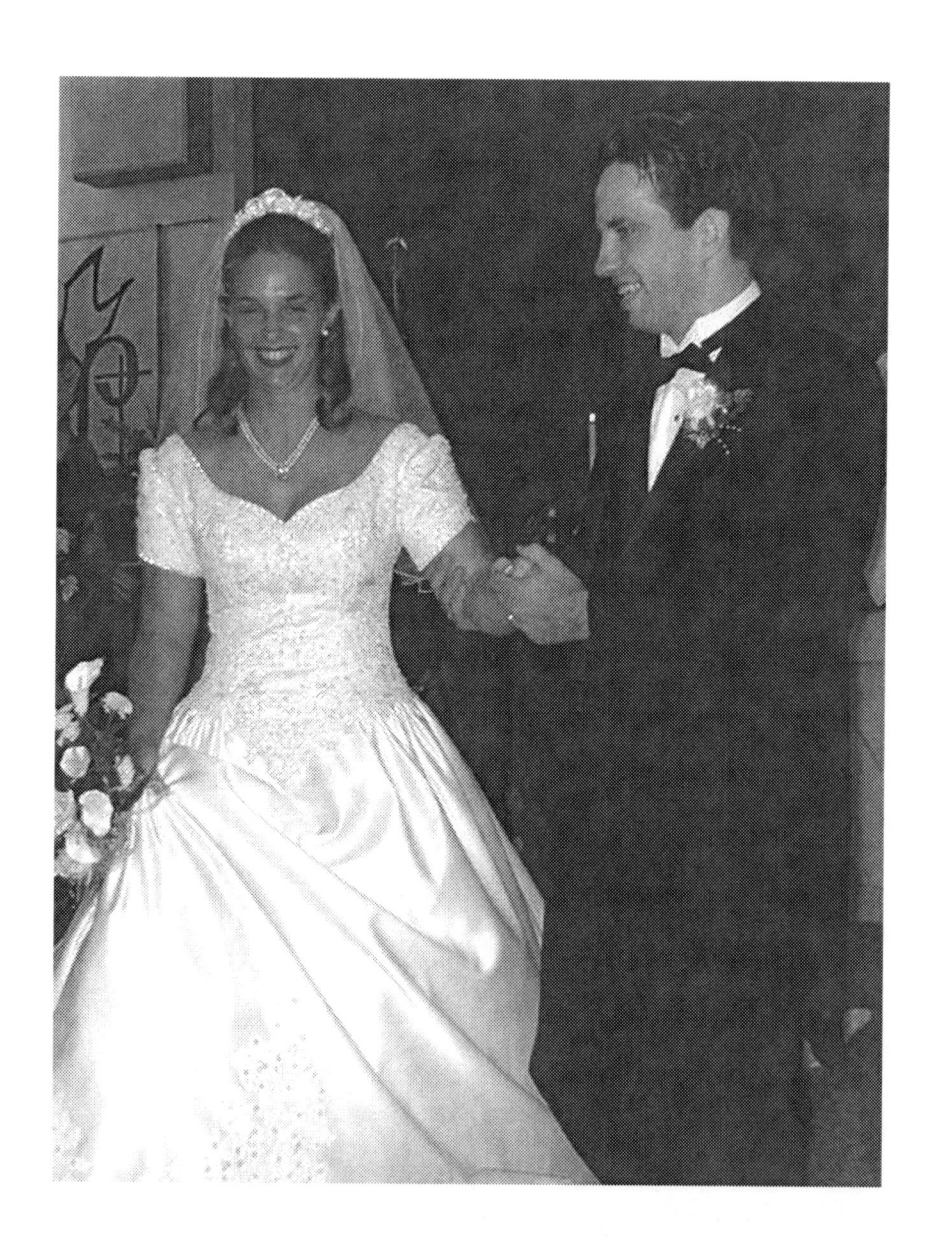

A Bright Day of Total Happiness After the Battle

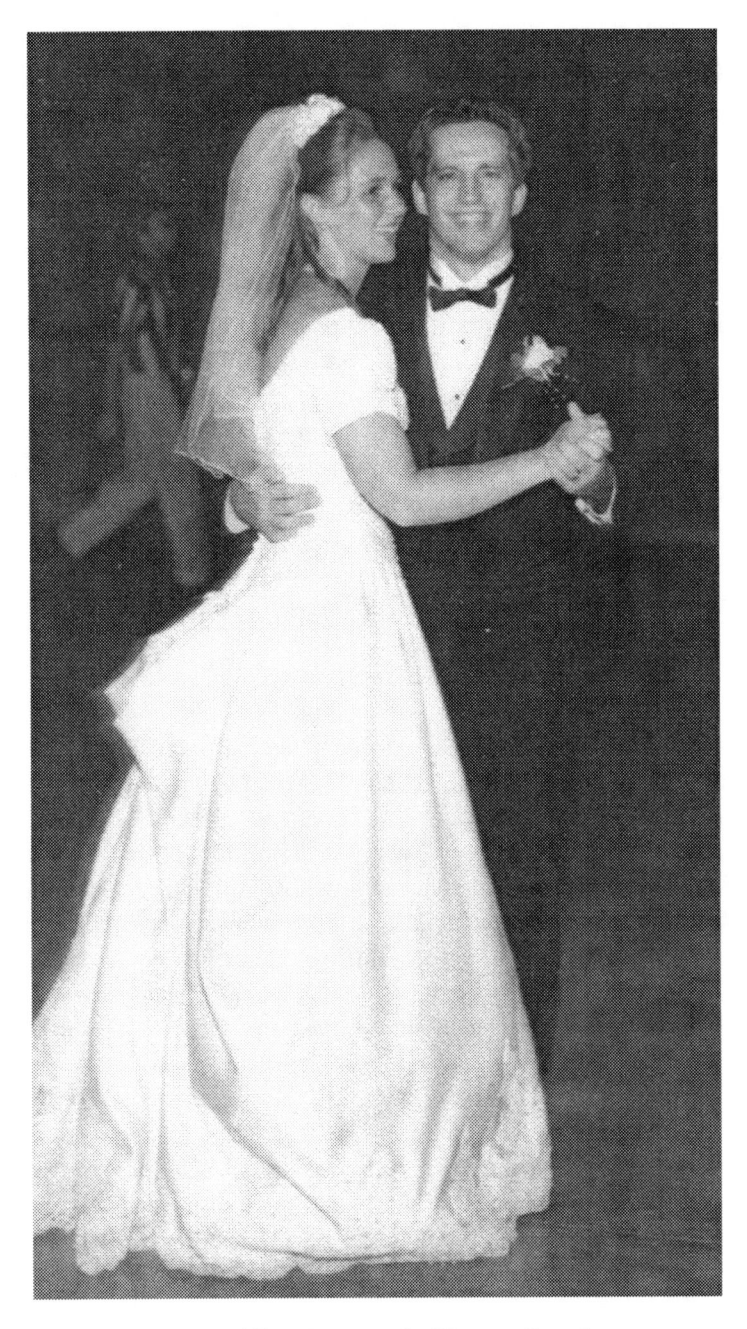

A Wedding Dance of a Happy Couple

Life was not the same as I had left it when I returned home. I knew it would probably soon be time to part ways.

I continued to keep in touch with my new friend Sue that I had met while Chad was in the hospital. Her husband got to return home for a short time and then went to a special care home. His cancer had spread too far by the time the doctors discovered it and they gave him no hope. My heart went out to her as she talked about and struggled with her emotions. Then I received the phone call from her to let me know that his cancer had won the battle. I called Chad to let him know. It was hard for him to express his sympathy though I could hear it in his tone of voice. He knew that it could have just as well been himself that had not survived.

Chad's counts returned to normal and he returned to work. The office he worked out of previously had no openings so he had to travel some distance each day to get to work. None the less he was glad to be back in society and working.

Everything seemed to be working out well and time was approaching for the wedding. As loose ends were tied up the wedding plans were falling into place.

The wedding was in St Louis, Missouri, where Rachael had been raised as a child. Her father was a minister so they would have him marry them in his church. I asked my fiancé to attend with me but he declined the offer. I packed the car and cruised down the interstate alone. Shawn and Cathy would be joining us later that day.

It was a fun and joyous time. It was the first time that any of the family, except for Tina, had seen Chad since before his diagnosis of leukemia. Most did not mention anything about what Chad had been through because they did not know how to approach it. A few family members did comment to me on how good he looked after going through what he had been through. I voiced my concerns of his appearance but they did not understand; they had not seen him when he was so ill. Upon seeing Chad again I felt uneasiness in my heart. He had regained his weight and much of his strength by this time. From a distance he looked to be back in good health.

I had seen Chad in his well days and his ill days and felt something was not quite right. To me his skin had an off color, a little yellowish cast. Looking into his eyes I saw a dull matte appearance I had seen before. There were few signs of brightness and clarity of the sparkle. I inquired of him how he was feeling. Still he assured me he was feeling good. By his actions you could not tell anything was wrong. He was happy and feeling blessed by the day's events.

The afternoon before the wedding all the wedding party got checked in at our hotels. We all met at the formal men's store so the men could get their tuxedos. Once that was done we all took a tour of a beer factory and then out to eat. Chad was holding up well and seemed to have plenty of energy.

The rehearsal and supper that evening went well and was fun. Chad refused to show any signs of tiredness around the events. My nephew's wife, Melissa, and I made an awful-looking bouquet out of silk flowers for Rachael to carry during the rehearsal. Over the past several family wedding rehearsals this had become sort of a tradition that we carried out for brides-to-be of the family. It was usually Tina and I who did this but her and Danny had not arrived yet. Chad and Rachael set up candles on the church alter that had Hawaiian dancers in grass skirts on them. Laughter was once again found after his battle as Chad was back to his outgoing humorous self.

After the supper several of the wedding party members and their spouses all met in the two double connecting rooms I had gotten at the hotel. There was much laughter as games and drinking took place. If Chad was tired he never let it show. He was enjoying sharing this special time with family and friends that he loved so dearly.

The day of the wedding arrived and several of us women met at the rehearsal hall to decorate. Rachael commented to me that she thought it was really special that Chad's grandmother and her grandmother were working together on decorating the tables. As soon as the decorating was done we returned to the hotel so that we all could prepare to get cleaned up to go to the church.

As I was preparing for the wedding Rachael called me at the hotel and asked me to stop and pick up a single long-stemmed white rose on my way to the church. She did not want a full bloom or a tightly closed bud. I thought it was for her to give me during the ceremony as I had seen that done at several weddings.

Arriving at the church I went to the room in the basement where she and the bridesmaids were dressing for the ceremony. I showed her the rose I had found and she said it was exactly what she wanted. She then asked me to go place it on the alter for her in memory of her departed mother. Tears filled my eyes as I felt honored. She could have asked her father or brother to do this task for her but instead she selected me to bestow this precious meaning. At that point I felt some of her loss of not having her mother there.

Soon the wedding ceremony began. As the ceremony took place a few tears leaked from my eyes. I was happy to see this day but they were not tears from my happiness. Chad and Shawn looked so handsome and I was so proud of them but they were not tears of an overwhelmed mother. Rachael looked absolutely beautiful and glowed that day but they were not tears of seeing her. I had cried those tears the day I went with her to try on wedding dresses. I cried to think that I was sitting in the church on this very day watching Chad get married. This day very easily was almost replaced by a funeral instead of a wedding for my son. They were tears of thankfulness and of feeling ever so blessed that my family was still three and soon to be four.

The wedding went well and was beautiful. Pictures were taken after the ceremony and everyone departed from the church. Family and friends then convened to a hall in the park for the reception. There was a promenade of the wedding party, a catered meal, the cake was cut, toasts were made and the dance started. Chad and Rachael had selected the song "What a Wonderful World" for the parent/child dance. What an appropriate choice for that moment after all that had happened. I was so proud and thankful to be living that moment. As we moved slowly across the dance floor I told him how proud I was of him and how glad I was that he selected such a wonderful woman to bring into our little family.

The day after the wedding several of us met at a restaurant for breakfast and then the newlyweds were off to Cancun, Mexico, for their honeymoon. I knew I would see them again in twenty days in Atlanta. A bone marrow biopsy was scheduled for June 26th. I would be by Chad's side to either celebrate his continued remission or cry with him if the leukemia had returned.

Even though my fiancé would not go to the wedding with me he did agree to drive out to Atlanta with me. My credit cards had maxed out and my bank funds were almost depleted so a drive was in order. This was of some concern but did not worry me too much as it was a small price to pay to be with my son to help him physically and emotionally. I just knew that God would somehow meet my needs. For after all, Chad was now still alive.

Plans were to return back to Kansas after a four-day visit. It was a road trip with a hope in my heart that we could make things better between us again. I felt all that time together in the car would reunite the closeness we had lost. We made stops at the Superman Museum in Metropolis, Illinois, at the Grand Ole Opry in Nashville, Tennessee, and Rock City in Chattanooga, Tennessee, on the way to Atlanta to make some memories. All seemed to be going well as we talked and laughed and enjoyed each other's company

In Nashville I started having problems with my car. Then there was another delay on the interstate. Just south of Nashville there was massive traffic congestion and we were detained in traffic for five hours before we were back into a steady flow of traffic. I prayed for my car to get us to Atlanta in time for me to go with Chad for his doctor's appointment. I could not bear the thought of him hearing any bad news alone and if it was good news I wanted to be by his side to celebrate.

The day was getting late and we were becoming tired. After a short stop at a rest area to get a few hours sleep we arrived in Atlanta the early morning the day before the appointment was scheduled that would tell us of the results of the bone marrow biopsy.

Chapter 11
June 2002

Understanding

If you could know the pain I feel
Would you understand
It is not pretend, it is for real
I just want you to hold my hand
If you could live the life I live
Would you understand
That each day is as if a sieve
And each moment a grain of sand
If you could know the hurts my heart aches
Would you understand
How many times one heart can break
As ones soul walks on this land
If you could count the tears I have cried
Would you understand
Not showing the tears I hide
Holding them back on my demand
If you would lose all that I have lost
Would you understand
All that my living has cost
In my shoes would you dare to stand
If you could trade places with me
Would you understand
Then you would feel and see what I feel and see
And then you would understand

I was excited when we pulled into the driveway. I was curious as to how Chad was feeling since his appearance had been a concern to me at the wedding. We were met at the door with smiles and hugs.

It was heartwarming to hear Chad and Rachael tell of all their honeymoon adventures. They both enjoyed what Mexico had to offer in sights and entertainment. All sounded wonderful until Chad voiced that he had drank some of the water. At first I was very concerned but then remembered that he did have his immune system back. Of course being a mother, I reminded him that he had been to Mexico before and knew he should not drink the water. He said he had drank it before he even thought about it but did not drink that much. He was worried himself that it may cause him problems. I assured him that if it was going to that he would have seen some effects from it by that time.

Later that evening I spoke with Chad about my concerns of his appearance at the wedding. The pale eyes and yellowish complexion were still present. Chad confessed to me that before the wedding his gums had started bleeding again. This was one of the symptoms we knew from past experience that was not a good sign. Chad openly voiced his concerns that he felt the test results were not going to be good ones. I tried to verbally reassure him to think positive and that God answers prayers and does miracles. Deep in my heart I felt a heaviness as I spoke. With his appearance and symptoms I knew there was a good chance the leukemia had returned also. I prayed hard that night for Chad to still be in remission and that God had passed this cup over him.

The next morning Chad and I drove to the doctor's office with much anticipation. My fiancé and Rachael remained at the house as she had much to do since their return from the wedding and honeymoon. We were not long in the waiting room before the nurse stepped to the door and called Chad's name. We were then escorted to a small room where we knew the routine well. Chad's vital signs were taken along with some blood work drawn and then he was weighed. After completion we were taken to an exam room to wait for the doctor.

Chad and I sat in the small exam room in silence. He sat in the chair against the back wall facing the door as if preparing to run if needed. I seated myself on the chair on the side wall between him and the door. I gave a few reassuring words that seemed to drop on deaf ears and fall to the hard tile floor. Five minutes passed and the doctor walked in and closed the door behind him. He sat down and opened the thick chart that he had carried in. After a short exchange of greeting he went right to the reason we were there: test results.

His smile diminished from his face and was replaced with a soberness that did not mean good results. Chad and I gave each other glances of fear and anticipation.

The words that followed lay heavy on our hearts even today. The biopsy results showed that the leukemia had returned. Tears welled in our eyes and ran down our cheeks as the doctor handed us each a box of facial tissues. We had so hoped and prayed so hard for this not to be the news we would hear.

The doctor then reviewed all that Chad had been through and his option of a bone marrow transplant. First Chad would have to go through more chemotherapy to see if they could get him back in remission so that he could even have a transplant. Maybe I missed something during conversations, but I do not think I did. I did not recall anyone telling us or reading anything about having to be in remission before having a bone marrow transplant. Chad would have to go through three more rounds of chemotherapy to his dismay.

Once again anger and fear controlled our lives. The battle was not over; it was just beginning again. It sucked, it wasn't fair, he was too young for this and why hadn't God answered my prayers? Again I reached for faith but it was hard to obtain sitting there at that moment. Once again anger and pain filled our hearts. In my mind I had so felt that through all the prayers and my faith the report would be good. Now I could not ignore the telltale signs I had seen at the wedding before the doctor's appointment and the knot I had felt in my stomach.

New plans were now set into place. Chad would return to the transplant specialist he had visited with previously when he had decided between the chemotherapy and bone marrow transplant. The two specialists would work together to get Chad into remission again and start preparing his body for the transplant.

As we left the clinic and got in the car Chad sat slumped heavily in the seat. He reached for his cell phone and placed a call to Rachael to tell her the unwelcome news. I asked him if he wanted to wait until we got to the house to tell her in person. He wanted to let her know right away and would not have to see the pain and disappointment on her face when she heard the news. I understood. It was hard enough for him to be handling the just heard news right now himself. With anger in his voice and tears in his eyes he told her what we had been told. My heart ached listening to him talk to Rachael. My heart felt heavy as I could sense the sadness and pain she was feeling with his every word. I wanted to take this burden from him and place it upon myself at any cost even though I was afraid of death itself.

I spoke with my fiancé when we got back to the house. I informed him that I could not return to Kansas because they would start the chemotherapy in two days. We scheduled him a flight out of Atlanta to return to Kansas for the following day. As I stood and watched him go through airport security I knew that this was the end of our relationship. He could not handle me being away for such long intervals for Chad's chemotherapy treatments so I knew our relationship would not survive Chad's bone marrow transplant. I would be signing on as the primary care provider, which meant I would be there for possibly up to a year or longer. I understood where his feelings were coming from and agreed.

Chad, Rachael and I now felt that we were starting all over again at square one as we drove to the hospital. Chad felt that all those other times of receiving chemotherapy and infections were something he could have avoided. Chad would be getting the first dose of chemotherapy to try and get him back into remission. This time they would try a different kind of chemotherapy called Mitozantrone with VP-16. We did not know how Chad's body was going to react to this new drug. We did not know if the medications they used to keep him comfortable before would even work with this type of chemotherapy. We could only hope and pray. Yes, even in our disappointment I still hung on to my faith. After all, Chad did make it through some near-death times and into remission previously. I did not want to take a chance that faith and prayers had something to do with that and I would not apply it again.

It was back to the unwelcome and all-too-familiar routine. Three days of chemotherapy treatments then five to seven days later there would be another hospital stay due to neutropenic fever and infection possibilities. I got into the habit of packing my suitcase the evening of day four once Chad was released from chemotherapy.

One week after chemotherapy Chad once again awoke in the middle of the night with a fever and vomiting. I called the doctor knowing we were heading back to the hospital. This time the doctor called for Chad's immediate admission into the hospital so we did not have to go through the emergency room. We were ever so thankful for that.

In a short time admissions had Chad assigned to his room and we were on our way up to the fifth floor to get him settled in. Smiles and hugs from the nursing staff greeted us.

Chad went through the same side effects from the new chemotherapy with the nausea, pain, loss of appetite, sores in his mouth and throat, loss of strength and being neutropenic. To some relief the nursing staff now had him as comfortable as possible with medications. What medications worked before was working now. There was question if the blood infection had returned so the infectious disease specialist was asked to come check Chad over. He was a very knowledgeable doctor but seemed to lack good bedside manner and appeared to be a very cold uncaring person. He was very matter of fact and then out the door.

With his admissions to the hospital Chad would miss their Boston terrier, Mattie. I found and purchased a large stuffed dog for Chad that looked like a real dog with glass eyes that appeared to be watching you. It was sitting on the chair in the corner of the room when the infectious disease specialist entered the room. He spotted the dog immediately as he entered the room and kept looking over at it. After examining Chad he went over and picked up the dog and sat down on a chair. Putting the stuffed dog on his lap, he started petting it as he talked with us. His tone of voice seemed to soften and he didn't seem rushed anymore. He let us know that he would be starting Chad on a new antibiotic for his infection. After the doctor left Chad and I looked at each other in puzzled amazement. We were both shocked and pleased to see that the doctor was human with feelings that he usually kept hidden. We had gotten to see a glimpse into that part of his world.

The stuffed dog became quite a novelty. As the medical staff members would enter the room for the first time since the dog arrived they would think we had brought a real dog in when they took first glimpse on it. I never thought that a stuffed animal would be such a conversation piece to liven up dull days. Chad marveled at teasing people about the dog and watching their reactions when they would enter the room.

The Fourth of July was upon us again only to find us again celebrating it at the hospital. The Fourth of July race through Atlanta was more exciting to watch than it was the previous year. Chad's nurse and newfound friend Elizabeth and her friend let Chad and I know that they were going to be in the race. I went out and watched with excitement of spotting them amongst the thousands of people that raced down the streets of Atlanta. I did see them and they waved and acknowledged my cheering them on. I reported back to Chad in his room as he had requested. I took pictures with a digital camera so that he could get to see them also.

Chad was given permission to go up to the top floor of the hospital family room that evening so that he could watch the fireworks. Once adorned in mask and two gowns he, Rachael and I rode the elevator for our Fourth of July celebration. It gave him a very small sense of being in touch with the outside world.

As we watched the fireworks they just did not seem to be as bright or beautiful as I had seen them in past years. I kept looking over at Chad sitting there with a mask on, wearing his hospital gowns with a pole beside him that was holding IV's that fed constantly into his veins. I had to fight back the tears.

I can still picture vividly the scene. For a little while Chad stood next to Rachael with the IV pole between them and I could see them and their reflection in the window against the flashes of color from the fireworks. Chad had lost all his hair again but had on his colorful Jamaican beret that he enjoyed wearing. He was also wearing a mask, two hospital gowns (one over the front and one over his backside) and the IV tubing that led from the hanging bag to the port in his chest.

As I videotaped the scene my thoughts became negative thinking of how, if Chad did loose his battle with leukemia, this would be some of the most precious videos in the world to me. I quickly cleared the negative thoughts from my mind and leaned on my faith of his recovery and thankfulness that he was with us right now. I looked at the two of them with loving eyes and a warm heart. I thought how God had selected the perfect person to stand by his side and love him. Rachael's strength was to be admired.

Ah yes, I had found another thing to be thankful for in all this craziness. Rachael was as strong and as stubborn as I was at that young age. To make it through this endeavor I knew that it was a good trait for her to have. She too had a tendency to cry her tears for Chad in silence, thinking she had to also be the strong one. We tended to reassure each other but not let the other see the tears. I look back now and think that we should have so that we could have comforted and supported each other a little better. We were both just scared and wanted to be the strong one and both stubborn enough to not let the other person know.

As we were in the elevator returning to the fifth floor Chad commented that if we spent one more Fourth of July at the hospital that it would have to become a tradition. I asked him why. He explained that if we do something three times in a row it becomes a tradition. That meant that we would always have to celebrate the Fourth of July at the hospital if we were there the following year. We all laughed out loud but on the inside prayed it not to be so.

After our ten-day stay and three chemotherapy treatments, Chad's doctor came in ready to release him to go home. The doctor recommended that he do what needed to be done to bank sperm to retain his sperm. He explained that with the bone marrow transplant there would be 98% chance that it would kill all viable sperm. Odds showed that seldom did viability ever return. Chad was on a tight time frame due to the leukemia being back and had to move quickly. He recommended where Chad was to go and suggested that he make the appointment immediately. Upon calling he was able to go in the following day. It could very well be his only chance to have offspring of his own.

In the past I had always thought that test tube, so to speak, babies were not what God intended. Now the thought of Chad and Rachael someday being able to have their own children or none at all opened my eyes to the miracle of science. I would no longer be so strongly opinionated to medical discoveries. I was thankful for God giving the knowledge to these doctors to make this even possible.

After a good night's sleep we drove to the sperm bank office. At first I felt a little uncomfortable sitting in the waiting room knowing what Chad was doing in the office. The uneasiness changed to calmness when I reminded myself of why this was so important. I am sure that Chad felt even more uncomfortable than I. When he returned to the waiting room I acted as if he had been in for a dentist appointment in hopes of making him feel more at ease. Neither of us said anything about it and went back to the house. We had to wait a few days for the sperm to be tested to make sure all was okay since he was no longer in remission. The report came back good so Chad returned one more time.

I was glad to know that in time there would be a little Chad in our lives. I was upset with myself when my mind drifted to thinking that if Chad was not a survivor to the leukemia battle that at least we would have a part of him to bring back into the world. I pondered on the fact of fear that they may have a child and then if Chad did not survive Rachael may move back to St Louis and take the child with her making it difficult for me to see her/him. I shivered at the thoughts I was having and got mad at myself for thinking such things. I reminded myself of my faith and trust in God and changed my thinking onto something else. I prayed that the next bone marrow biopsy that would take place soon would come back clean of any cancer cells.

Chapter 12
August 2002

Do Dreams Come True

Dreams are of beauty and joy
For every person, girl or boy
They can set a goal for you
And sometimes even dreams come true

With skies of blue and birds singing
In a distance a church bell is ringing
Peaceful times to recall to mind
Calming head and heart I try to find

Sometimes dreams can ache inside
For within yourself you cannot hide
Wants and needs that may never be
That only in your eyes you see

Perhaps someday, dreams may stop
Because like a balloon they can quickly pop
With heavy heart and tear-filled eyes
Have your dreams been telling you lies

With lack of hope you cease to try
After awhile you do not even cry
Everything falls down at your feet
And you feel you no longer can compete

Just as all seemed to be getting better a new problem reared its ugly head in Chad's battle. Chad had found a mass in one of his testicles. A new doctor's face now appeared to join the fight, a surgeon. During a visit to his office tests were run along with an examination. First the doctor wanted to see if the chemotherapy would dissolve the mass and then they would decide if surgery was really necessary. To our delight the chemotherapy dissolved the mass but still the surgeon felt strongly about removal. It was decided that it was in Chad's best interest to have the testicle removed. There was some reluctance but the doctor appeared to be very sure of his decision. I backed him and reassured Chad that he would be no less a man.

Sue called that she wanted to come to Atlanta to be support for us during Chad's surgery. Even after the loss of her husband she wanted to be kept up on how Chad was doing. She and her daughter-in-law came to sit with me while Chad was in surgery. It was nice to have a friend close by. She and her daughter-in-law had driven one-hundred-fifty miles to come be with us. The surgery went well and Chad was on his way to recovery. My supporters departed to return home so that I could sit in the recovery room at Chad's bedside with him.

After the biopsy results came back from the surgery we were informed that there was still cancer cells found in the tissue that was removed. We were thankful for the decision to remove the testicle.

During Chad's recovery stay in the hospital the doctors decided that this was a good time to put Chad through a battery of tests. The doctors wanted to make sure there was no other cancer hiding itself. There was a CAT scan, ultrasound, breathing tests, body x-rays, an echocardiogram, blood work, MRI and a spinal tap to check fluids and insert chemotherapy into his spine to replace the fluid they had removed. All this was very tiring and stressful for Chad. There was not an inch on the outside or inside of Chad's body that had not been poked and tested. After about a week he was finally released to return home.

During this time I took a few afternoons and went to get my car checked out to see what the problem was. Rachael was going to be able to be home with Chad. I found out that there seemed to be a problem with the transmission. Considering the cost and comfort for Chad I opted to find another vehicle. My car was a convertible and it was not comfortable for Chad to lie down in on our trips to and from the hospital when he was not feeling well. My search led me to an SUV. Chad would now be able to ride more comfortably and have more than enough room if he needed to lie down.

In August it was time for another bone marrow biopsy to see if the chemotherapy had worked to get Chad's body back into remission. I hated to see Chad go through another biopsy, as he had had so many already. Yet we were all anxious to find out if the chemotherapy had done its job and gotten Chad back into remission.

The results we received from the biopsy were good, no cancer cells detected. In all our joy and relief of the good test results I thought about the long hard road Chad still had ahead of him and the mountains that still needed to be moved. I prayed for him to have the strength both physically and emotionally to continue with his long journey.

With Chad back home and life as close to normal as could possibly be, it was again time for me to depart for a short while. We knew that it would take some time for them to put Chad through all the tests and for them to find a bone marrow donor. I knew I would need to return to Kansas and begin preparing for a very long stay with my next visit.

Once again I would be on my way back to Kansas to return to the life I had left behind so many times before. It seemed like a long drive alone but gave me much time to think and make plans. This time I knew that the next time I returned to Georgia it could be for up to a year. Returning the next time meant placing personal items in storage and moving to Georgia for an undetermined length of time.

Arrangements had been started to begin preparations for the bone marrow transplant before I had even left. Chad would have a short time for him and Rachael to have some personal time before their lives were totally turned upside down and sideways again.

Chad reminded me on occasion that he could not have the bone marrow transplant without me staying with him through the entire process. He questioned me as to if I really wanted to dedicate up to a year of my life taking this task on. Needless to say I had no second thoughts about doing it.

I was designated as the primary care provider for Chad. The transplant would not be done if I did not sign a paper with the Bone Marrow Transplant Clinic stating that I would be there to care for him seven days a week/twenty-four hours a day. At no time was Chad to be allowed to be by himself until completely released by the doctor after transplant and treatments. Rachael was also asked to sign on as a primary care provider for when I may need to be absent. She also gave no hesitation.

We all enjoyed a wonderful evening together. The following morning I and cat Whiskers loaded up and headed out. The trip back to Kansas was good but the road seemed long.

Now I had to move on with my life. I kept busy with working my job and preparing for the move. Shawn decided to remain in the apartment we had been living in so I did not have to put too much into storage. Many things I would leave for him to use.

When I returned to work everyone was glad to see me and anxious to hear about how Chad was doing. I also received a most welcome surprise. I was informed that other employees of our employer all across the United States were giving up some of their vacation days to me. What this meant was that I would still receive a few paychecks to financially help me with expenses to help get through this time. I was much relieved as by this time I had maxed out three credit cards with flying back and forth from Kansas to Georgia, helping with Chad's medications and medical expenses and helping Chad and his fiancée make ends meet. Truly this was a blessing.

Another financial break came when I went to visit my great uncle. He informed me that it was in his heart to help me financially. I informed him that I would do okay and he did not need to help me in any way except with emotional support. He would not hear of it. He wanted to help with this hardship for Chad and me. I told him that it was not necessary and if he could just be there to guide Shawn during my absence that would be enough. He still insisted.

Soon the call came from Chad that they were ready to start preparing him for the transplant. He also reminded me that I would have to sign a paper stating that I would remain with him as his primary care provider for the full length of time that could be up to a year. He reminded me that I had the option of making such a commitment also. I knew that there would be no transplant if I did not sign the paper so there was no question in my mind what I needed to do. I knew that if I did not sign this paper there would be no Chad.

I went in to inform my boss that I would be leaving the next day. He informed me that he would need me to stop in the morning and see him before I left town. He would not say why at that time. I was guessing that he was going to tell me that I would be gone for too long of a time this time and they would need to replace me at my job.

The next morning I prepared to leave and say my goodbyes. I placed my final bags in the car along with my pet carrier containing Whiskers. I stopped by my place of work on the way out of town as instructed by my boss. To my surprise all the employees in the office had fixed up a care box for me. There was food, personal items, boxes of tissues, and an envelope for me. Tears filled my eyes as I opened the envelope and found it full of money. I could not believe my eyes. I told them they did not have to do that. I was told that they knew I would need money to get a motel room and eat on the way back to Atlanta. There was enough money in the envelope that when I returned to Atlanta I could even buy some of Chad's medications for him that he needed. Leaving my workplace and dear friends I headed down interstate 70 to make my move east.

Chapter 13
November 2002

When Enough Is Enough

When you no longer want to be
When you want to run and flee
Look up to the sky
When teardrops are in your eye
When your mind is all confused
And you are feeling that you have been used
When your heart is heavy and sad
A pull between hurt and mad
When everything seems to go wrong
Making the day seem oh so long
When answers cannot be found
And you feel you are losing ground
When all hope seems lost
Unable to get it back, at any cost
When your back is against the wall
And then you start to fall
When you have lost all courage and fight
And you cannot see any light
When your body is tired and weak
And you cannot be anything but meek
When teardrops on your pillow want to drop
Because you feel you are a total flop
When you want to scream "that is enough"
And you want so badly to be tough
When you feel there is nothing you can do

HOLDING ON FOR DEAR LIFE

Look in the mirror at you
Ask yourself "You are who?"
Who are you being harmful to?
Then you will see a brand new you
Pick yourself up, dust yourself off and
Remember you are in God's hand.

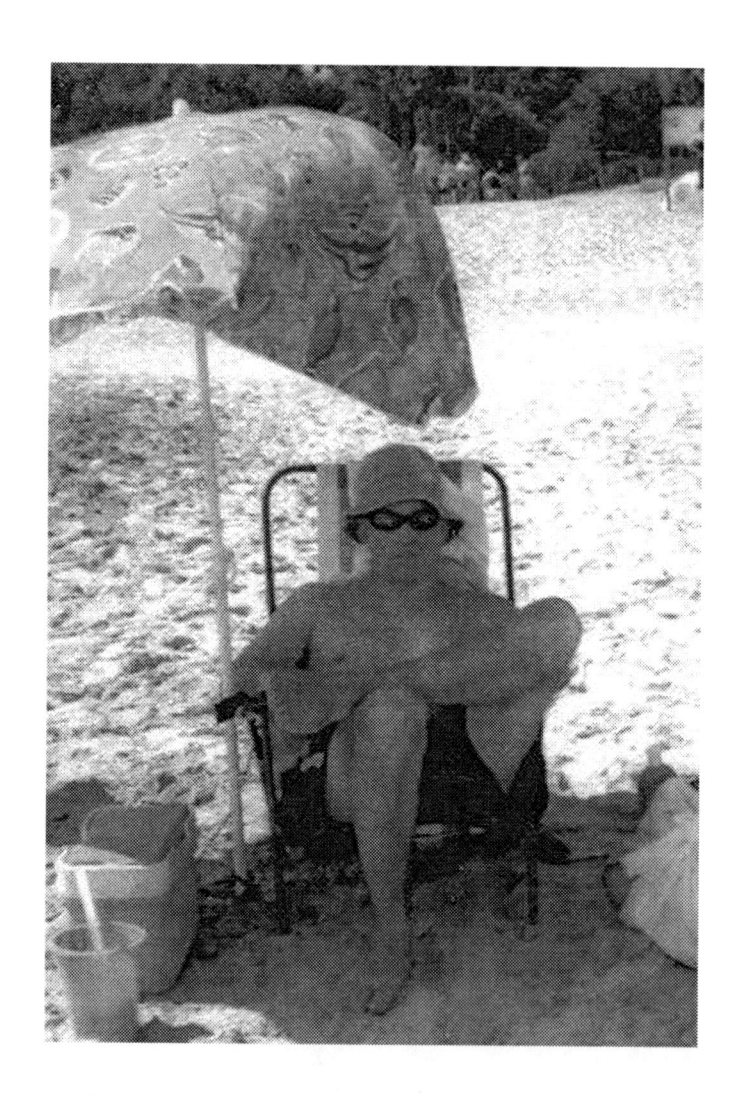

A Favorite Place to Be
A Place of Calm Serenity

When I arrived preparations were well under way for the bone marrow stem cell transplant. There was not a square inch on Chad's body that was not once again scanned, x-rayed, poked and prodded. Three full days of rigorous testing made Chad weak and exhausted.

Since there were no compatible donors available from family they began the process to try and use Chad's own stem cells for his transplant. He was placed in a private room in the clinic and connected to a large machine. He was advised that he would feel very cold and the procedure would last about four hours. During the process his blood was pumped through the machine and the stem cells were separated out and went into an intravenous bag. They would then take them and "wash" them to remove any that were cancer cells and leave only the healthy cells to return to him. This procedure was attempted three times with little success. Not enough healthy cells could be collected to produce enough for a transplant.

The medical staff now turned to the national transplant donor list to try and find a match for Chad. They would need to find someone that would have all ten antigens that Chad's body would need to accept. There was a reality that his body could reject donor cells and it would kill him. It would be a foreign substance introduced into his body and his body may reject it.

Success at finding a donor for a match was looking pretty doubtful. When Chad's work-up was done they discovered that he had a rare antigen in his blood. His father and I were asked to sign releases to give blood so that it could be used to help with the medical research about this antigen. When all seemed hopeless for a transplant we were informed that they had finally found two donors that were compatible enough out of all the thousands of donors on the registry. We now had new hope and uplifted spirits.

My parents had been wanting to come out for a visit to see Chad before he had the transplant. My older sister called me about her and her son coming out and bringing our mother and father with them. I thought it to be a most wonderful idea and Chad was very excited.

On December fifth my oldest sister, Carolyn, and her son, Craig, arrived for a visit. With them they brought my parents. Chad was overwhelmed with happiness to have family come out for a visit. It helped to reassure him that he had a lot of support in his battle. He marveled at the fact that there were now other men in the house besides himself.

Carolyn had also been a blessing to me for support and understanding. In the past, two of her sons had been in a traffic accident that almost took their lives away. She understood most of the feelings I was trying to cope with.

During their stay we toured a few of the local museums and had a wonderful visit. My mother, sister and I decorated a large Christmas wreath for Chad and Rachael to hang on their front door for the holiday season. Chad thought it was wonderful and voiced how much it meant to him. Rachael was very pleased with it and proud to hang it on their front door.

All too soon it was time for their departure and for Chad to move forward with the preparations for his transplant. It was difficult to see them leave. I so wished they could have stayed longer but understood their need to return home. For some time even after they left, Chad still had an upbeat spirit.

Since the donor had been located and agreed to donating stem cells, the doctors could begin to prepare Chad for his transplant. The date for transplant was scheduled for December 12th. What a wonderful early Christmas present this was going to be. At this time we had no idea how intense, difficult and painful it was going to be for Chad to be prepared for such a procedure.

Chad would once again go through another regimen of chemotherapy so the doctors could make sure that all cancer cells were dead in his body. Chemotherapy was also inserted into his spine via a spinal tap so if there were any cancer cells there they would be killed. It was explained to me that any chemotherapy he received intravenously would not be able to go into his spinal fluid.

Again Chad was dealing with nausea, vomiting, pain and loss of appetite and strength. Again we would be facing the fears of no immune system. We were told that after the transplant Chad's immune system would return quickly.

I was instructed by the doctor to keep a daily log beginning five days before transplant and for the next one-hundred days after transplant. At the time I wondered why but soon it made sense to me as those days passed. Each day seemed to run into the next at a massive state of speed and events. Each day was different with many changes.

The fifth day before transplant Chad received more chemotherapy and came home with a portable IV pump with medication that would protect the lining of his bladder against medications and radiation that he would be receiving.

After his visit to the clinic the following morning, we had to go over to the radiation department at the hospital. A body form was made for Chad as he would have to lie in a certain position and not move during his total body radiation treatments. There were certain parts of the body that could not handle such intense radiation. It was described to me as having his insides in a microwave oven. However, they would have to monitor very accurately how much radiation he received. The form was made of plastic and foam.

That evening Chad voiced his anxiety and fear about not knowing if his body would accept or reject the transplant donor's cells and about getting total body radiation treatments. I could not even imagine what he was going through in his mind yet alone his body. He was much too young to have to be going through all this. Once again I thought of how brave he was to be doing this. It made me angry that he should have to be dealt such a dreadful endeavor. He was such a joy to everyone's life that he encountered. We talked in deep length that night and gave each other a long hug before retiring for the night.

That night as I lay in the still darkness I came up with an idea to remove this large mountain in a physical as well as mental way. I got a piece of shiny gold construction poster board. Using markers I made a sun with a rainbow under it. Under the rainbow I wrote "U R OUR HERO." I cut out boulders from shiny silver poster board and placed small ones at the top and large ones at the bottom and placed them in the shape of a mountain attaching them with Scotch tape onto the gold board.

The next morning I explained to Chad that each day he would remove one boulder from the mountain to tear it down. From the large boulder there were six boulders marked with chemo, eight boulders marked radiation and one bolder at the bottom marked transplant. Behind those boulders were more small boulders marked from one to one-hundred to represent each of the one-hundred days after transplant. I placed it on the side of the refrigerator so he would pass by it as he came in the back door of the house when he would come in after appointments. He got to remove the first five chemo boulders at that time.

The fourth day before transplant Chad completed his last chemotherapy treatment at the clinic. The first thing Chad did when he got home was to remove the last chemo boulder from his mountain. He did well the rest of the day but was starting to feel weak and tired. It seemed to help put everything he was going to go through in a material form. He could then see his accomplishments and see the number of things he had to go through dwindle down.

Day three of countdown they started the first total body radiation treatment. Chad seemed calm but I knew he was feeling much anxiety. He wanted me to go back with him but we were informed that I had to wait in the waiting room. Chad was taken back to the radiation room as I waited anxiously in the waiting area. The nurse came out to tell me that Chad voiced his concerns of getting nauseated from the treatments. She suggested that Chad take his medication for anxiety each morning before going in for treatments.

After the completion of the first radiation treatment we went over to the clinic where Chad had blood work drawn. It showed his potassium was low. It was low enough that he had to have one IV bag of potassium and two potassium tablets. His magnesium was also low so he had to have one IV bag with magnesium in it.

Once we finally finished with the medical regimen we returned home where Chad went to his bedroom and lay down to rest and cried. My heart was breaking for him. I tried to comfort him but did not feel that I was making much headway.

On the morning of day two Chad took his medication for anxiety along with his medication for radiation. Following the second radiation treatment we proceeded to the bone marrow clinic per our now normal protocol. His appointment at the bone marrow clinic again included IV fluids with potassium and magnesium. After completion of the IV therapy he took more medication for nausea and anxiety. He felt hungry and did manage to eat a few bites of a biscuit. Due to the previous radiation treatment he was feeling pain in his stomach and had a headache.

We proceeded back over to the hospital for his next radiation treatment, which would include his lungs this time. Chad seemed to feel some better after all the IV therapy so I was in hopes that the radiation would not be as hard on him this time. My hopes were not met. Returning him back home he became nauseated and started vomiting. He went straight to bed and asked me to take the boulder down from his mountain for that day. The remainder of the evening he had nausea, vomiting and complained of his body aching and a headache. There was very little sleep that night.

To my relief Tina flew in from Kansas to give support. It was a great comfort to see her. I knew I could let down my "brave one" guard around her and let loose of the tears and voice the fears I had been dealing with inside.

Day one of countdown brought another trip to the hospital and clinic with Chad fighting against nausea and vomiting. Radiation was first on the agenda for this day. Chad handled it fairly well.

After the radiation Chad was taken over to the bone marrow clinic for his appointment by wheelchair. He was just too weak and ill to make the trip on his own accord. Once at the clinic he was placed on a bed in a private room so that he could lie down and rest better. He was given IV medication for pain and for nausea. I was instructed that we were to alternate between his nausea/anxiety medication and a nausea medication every three to four hours but to watch for drowsiness and cut back if needed.

Once the IV fluids were completed we wheeled Chad back to the hospital for a second round of total body radiation. The nurse let Tina and I go with Chad to the radiation room. She showed us how they placed him in the form and how the radiation treatment was given. My heart felt heavy and tears were fought back as I watched Chad through the glass wall just outside the room as he went through the treatment. Once the treatment was completed Chad was taken to an exam room as the radiologist wanted to see him.

Chad now had sores in his mouth causing him discomfort, nausea, vomiting, an aching body, a headache and ulcers in his stomach. Tears welled in his eyes as he told me that this was worse than anything he had gone through with the chemotherapy. He began to cry and asked me to have them just stop everything. He said he would rather die than go through any of this anymore.

I tried to keep my tears at bay and give comforting words as I held him in my arms. Tina could not hold back her emotions and began to cry and stepped out of the room. Once I had Chad calmed down I told him I was going to step out to check on Tina but would be right back. I stepped out to check on her. I knew that she was feeling the pain as if Chad was her own flesh and blood. She also had two sons and we both felt as the other's children were just as much a part of our own. She stated that even though I had talked to her on the phone about all that had been going on it was not anything like being there and seeing it for herself. She was now a part of the reality that Chad, Rachael and I were facing with each passing day of this battle. She could not believe or could imagine how I had managed to hold myself together. I told her I did have my times of falling apart but that my faith in God to heal Chad was what I hung on to most. I did not want to give up the hope for his recovery but there were times of doubt.

The radiology specialist arrived to see Chad. Seeing the emotional and physical state Chad was in, the radiologist contacted Chad's transplant doctor. The two decided that it would be best for him to be put into the bone marrow transplant unit in the hospital where he could get the medications he needed through his IV port to keep him as comfortable as possible. I was relieved and glad to think he would soon be feeling some better even if he was sedated.

Chad was transported to the Bone Marrow Transplant Unit in the hospital. It was a very controlled environment. All the air in the unit was filtered air. The only drinking water was bottled water. Before entering the unit we were instructed on the procedure for entering and departing the unit. Through the first double doors was an anteroom. In there was where you adorned a long-sleeve gown and shoe covers. There were hooks to hang up any coat or jacket you may have that could not be taken past the second set of double doors. We were then instructed on the proper hand washing technique we were to use. It was time consuming but it was for the safety of Chad and all the other patients that were beyond the second set of double doors.

Chad had already been taken to his room and placed on his hospital bed. He looked fragile lying there. He was so close to transplant and he was so physically and mentally beaten that all I could do was try and comfort him and pray.

Chapter 14

A Call for Help

I need some help from you, dear Lord
Please show me what to do
I am restless and I am tired, Lord
I need some help from You

My feelings are so mixed up inside
I feel so down and blue
There is no one else in to confide
I know You have my answer too

Dear Lord, help me please this day
To find out just where I stand
Just let me know, if I may
I need someone to reach out a hand

I want to smile and be glad
Just like I used to be
My life is so messed up and sad
A sign from above, please send to me

Day zero (December 12th) had finally arrived and newfound hope was in sight. Day zero also meant two more rounds of total body radiation for Chad before the transplant. We were worried for Chad to survive all he would go through on this day yet anxious and excited that this was the day of possible new birth for him.

Chad did manage to make it though both treatments of radiation with the help of medication to keep him as comfortable as possible and partly sedated. Once the second treatment of radiation was completed we waited with anticipation to hear the word that the donor's stem cells were at the hospital.

Chad had asked the nurses and doctor frequently over the past two weeks about where they had found the donor. By policy they are not allowed to tell us until one year after date of transplant. That did not stop Chad from asking even though he knew they would not tell him. On occasion he did like to bug people just for the heck of it.

Our first word came about seven-forty-five in the evening. The nurse came into Chad's room and informed us that they had just gotten word that the plane carrying the cells had arrived at the airport and it was en route to the hospital. Tina and I quietly voiced to each other that we had both thought of the fear of the transport being in an accident or held up in traffic due to an accident. After all we were talking of the cells being transported from the south side of Atlanta through downtown traffic on highway 75 to the north part of downtown Atlanta.

Chad seemed more nervous than ever though he was trying not to show it. I asked and he answered, "I know that if my body rejects the donor cells it could kill me." I searched for words to remind him that if they did not do the transplant he was definitely going to die; the cells were a chance at living.

Our next report brought much excitement and relief when at eight-thirty that evening we were told that the cells were in the hospital and were going through a final match with Chad's cells in the lab. Chad now seemed to show some excitement and a more positive attitude.

After a wait that seemed like forever we were told that the doctor and the stem cells were now in the bone marrow unit and they would be starting the transplant at eleven-thirty that evening. Only fifteen more minutes to wait.

In my mind I did not comprehend the severity of this procedure at that moment in time. Death could have been at the doorstep; a doctor had to be present during the procedure in the event of a reaction or death. The only thing my mind wanted to conceive was that Chad was now going to be able to have a chance to beat this battle with the help of a wonderful anonymous person.

The nurse arrived in the room with her transplant kit (an emergency kit so that if Chad's body started rejecting the donors cells) and also brought us a letter from the donor. She handed the envelope to Chad and he opened the envelope and took out the letter. Opening up the folds of the sheet of paper he began to read the first sentence. Upon hearing the first sentence we all began to cry. Chad handed me the letter and asked me to read it aloud for him and Tina to hear. Pausing briefly on occasion to gulp and catch my breath I read the letter. The donor told us that he was a middle-aged family man. He hoped that by making this donation he was giving a chance for Chad's life to continue. He also wanted to wish us all a Merry Christmas. There was not a dry eye within hearing distance of my voice.

The transplant was given through an IV. It was a cloudy yellow semi-thick consistency in a plastic bag that we had been waiting for. Who would have thought that this thing that could give us such hope and possible future life to Chad would be something so simple looking? In just a matter of about one and one-half hours later the transplant was completed. We had expected some major event to take place that was no more than like getting a unit of blood through an intravenous port. We were glad that it was that simple for Chad.

With Chad's anxiety level lowering because the infusion was done and with the medications they had given him, he now rested and went to sleep. He said he felt more relieved that the transplant was over and he had no reaction. His stress of the outcome from it at this time had finally subsided.

We had been told that if Chad's body rejected the donor cells that it could kill him and also that if he did not get graft versus host disease (GVHD) from the donor cells that that could kill him also. If he did get graft versus host disease and it could not be kept under control that could also kill him. Not a win-win situation by far. Yet we had no choice but to take the chances.

The following morning was now count-up, it was again day one. Chad had slept well through the night, as did Tina and I. We were all emotionally exhausted. Upon awaking Chad seemed to be relieved to see the daylight of a new day and that Tina and I were there by his side. He did complain of slight nausea and was medicated for that. He was given a dose of what they called "follow-up" chemotherapy, a dressing change to his IV port site on his chest and then he was discharged to go home from the hospital.

Before departing from the hospital I had left the transplant unit to go to the cafeteria for some breakfast. While in the anteroom I met a girl that her brother, Eric, had just had a bone marrow transplant the same day as Chad had had his. He was also around the same age as Chad. She was the donor for his transplant. With tears in my eyes I voiced to her of how she was just as much a hero as her brother. She gave him another chance at life. We shared emotions and particulars about Chad's and her brother's illnesses. Through shared tears we said our good-byes with a hug. Her brother was diagnosed with Hodgkin's disease and this was his second transplant because it had returned after two years of remission.

The medications that Chad was released from the hospital on could have filled a pharmacy shelf. We had a list of fifteen medications that we would be administering to him at various times of the day. A schedule was written out for us to follow with instructions that, depending on his counts and results of daily lab work, we would be changing frequently. Along with all these medications that he would be taking by mouth he would be getting intravenous medications through his port with our daily visits to the bone marrow clinic. During the one-hundred-day count these medications were daily but changed in dosage amounts frequently depending on results included the following:

Acyclovir, Compazine, Zofran, Loperamide, Ambien, Klor-Con, Spornox, Pepcid, Tequin, Paxil, Phenergan, Ativan, Oxycodone KCL, Chlorhexide Gluconate oral rinse, Swish&Swallow, Leucorin, Benadryl patches, Methotrexate, Neupogen, Prograf, Magnesium. Most of these medications were daily, some were one or more tablets, some were to be given more than once a day and some were only on specific days, others were as needed. It was a very tight regimen. I found out the second and most important reason as to why I was told to keep a notebook.

Chapter 15

What Do You Say

What do you say when your world falls apart
It is like a balloon being hit by a dart
All hope and dreams vanish into the air
It makes you wonder, "God, do you care?"
My God, have you forsaken me
All my pain do You not see
Take this burden away from me
I want to be alive and illness free
My Lord, do You not hear my cry
My Lord, I do not want to die

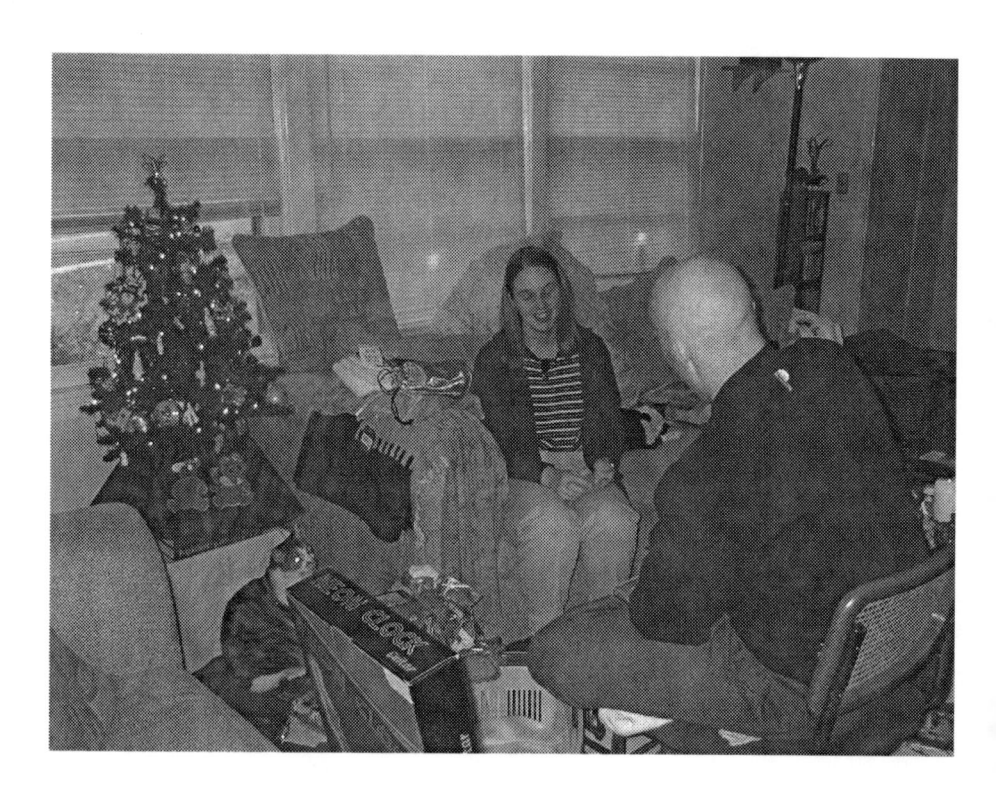

A Christmas Gift of Life

During the course of the first week after transplant it seemed that any kind of movement caused severe nausea. Even our daily trips to the clinic caused Chad to have nausea to the point of vomiting, which was treated with the Phenergan and Ativan and Compazine. If one of the medications did not work after four hours we would try the next one. Another frequent complaint was a headache, which was treated with Oxycodone. Chad tried to eat as well as possible but almost every time he ate he would be vomiting within the following half hour.

Tina returned back to Kansas on day three. It was such a comfort to have her by our side for that little extra moral support. God could not have sent me a better friend/sister-in-law. It was left to her shoulders to give report of the transplant events to family upon her return. She took a copy of the letter from the donor with her and read it aloud to our immediate family at their Christmas gathering. She reported back to me that there was not a dry eye by the time she completed reading it. This battle was affecting the lives of many.

Other symptoms arose that week including complaints of numbness in his hand to his elbow and a scratchy, sore throat. With the doctor's exams he could not explain the numbness of the hand and elbow. He recommended that Chad eat small amounts of food more often and drink lots of liquids. They also recommended trying a patch that was worn behind the ear to try and assist with the nausea from the car rides.

I kept a bag in the car for Chad for the times that he would become nauseated during the ride to and from the clinic. On one particular day he became nauseated as we were getting out of the Blazer. He did not have time to get the bag out from under the seat he was sitting on. He vomited inside the vehicle. He felt badly about doing this and apologized numerous times. I assured him that I was not upset and that it was not a big deal so not to worry about it. I know he still felt bad about it.

By the end of the week the patches seemed to be taking effect and helping with the nausea in connection with taking a nausea and an anxiety medication by mouth a half hour before leaving the house. The complaints still continued of mouth and throat pain, headache and sleeplessness. The doctor had Chad start taking a sleeping pill each evening to help him rest.

On day seven he was given a bag of platelets along with his regular daily IV medications. Chad despised those days that he had to receive platelets or blood; he knew it meant we would be at the clinic for at least eight hours. None of our visits were less than six hours. Comfort was not the best of conditions at the clinic but they did the best they could with recliners. There were small televisions to watch at each recliner. They also had a collection of movies that were available for anyone to watch.

Depending on the severity of Chad's symptoms he would occasionally be placed in a small room with a bed and a chair so that he could lie down. On days he felt better his boredom was relieved by napping, watching television or selecting a movie from the many VHS tapes that were available to select from out of the cabinet in the hallway. It was difficult trying to find a movie that Chad had not already seen after this long. One day as he was sleeping I went and arranged all the movies in alphabetical order. Everyone seemed pleased that I had taken the time to do that for them. It was short lived that they stayed that way, but gave me something to do. During this time Chad started watching the judge shows on television and was becoming hooked on them.

By day eight (December 20th) Chad began running a fever. We were noticing involuntary muscle jerks and some hand tremors. He was complaining of a stuffy nose, sore throat and was coughing. During his exam at the clinic that day they discovered he needed to have two units of blood along with his usual medications. The doctor explained that the jerks and tremors were expected because it was a side effect from one of the medications. I wish I had known that ahead of time so we could have alleviated some fear. As for the other symptoms, they recommended rotating between the Ativan and Compazine for the nausea, taking Oxycodone for the throat pain and to get some over the counter allergy/sinus medication for the stuffy nose.

By day eleven (December 23rd) there was still no relief from the symptoms and a new one arose. Chad noticed a rash on his chest and back. We were told that it was probably a sign of the GVHD (graft verses host disease). A new fear arose with the reminder that if not kept under control it could mean his death. A unit of platelets was given again. Transfusions of platelets and blood were now becoming a common thing, almost daily.

Departing the clinic that day Chad went home with a portable IV pump that contained Prograf that would help with any side effects of GVHD. This medication had to be monitored closely as it could cause problems with other organs in his body. I was instructed on what to do if the alarm went off on the portable IV pump and how to discontinue it.

Monthly respiratory treatments were started at this time. Chad was given a regimen of breathing capacity tests and then he was given a breathing treatment that he inhaled from a machine that had antibiotics in it.

It was not until Christmas Eve, day twelve, that a biopsy was done of the rash area to detect if it was GVHD or not. It was also the first day since transplant that Chad did not require a shot of Neupogen. He managed to keep down an oatmeal cream pie for breakfast and a peanut butter and jelly sandwich for lunch. Things were looking forward.

It had been difficult finding time to get out and find Christmas presents even though they would not be elaborate due to lack of funds. The joy of having Chad alive with us to celebrate was the only gift I needed. I did wish that Shawn and Cathy could have joined us but there were no funds left to bring them out to Georgia.

I did get time away from the house to shop usually on weekends. It was a break for me and gave Chad and Rachael a time without mother-in-law around. Rachael had placed decorations out and I had gotten some Christmas plaster pieces and paint and made a few decorations to set out also. Since we could not have live plants around the house it meant a real Christmas tree was out of the question. Rachael placed a small fake tree up in the living room and decorated it. It looked like Christmas around the house but it just did not have the excitement that should be with the season.

Christmas day started out with our usual trip to Chad's appointment. Since the Bone Marrow Clinic was closed for the holiday we were instructed to go to the Bone Marrow Unit in the hospital. While there, Chad got his daily blood work drawn and received his intravenous fluids. I was pleased to see that on this day Chad was starting to feel well enough that he started visiting with other patients who had also reported in for fluids.

Returning home Chad went to bed and took a nap. Once he awoke we opened gifts. It was a Christmas I will hold dear in my heart for the rest of my life. I will never forget the joy that filled my heart and the tears that welled in my eyes as I thanked God for one of the best Christmas presents I would ever receive in my lifetime. Chad was there to be a part of it. I was also informed by Chad and Rachael that they were going to start the process for an in vitro pregnancy. I was going to get to be a grandmother sometime during the next year if all went well.

Chapter 16
January 2003

Holding On for Dear Life

What is there left to say
I do not want to go away
I continue with the fight
Holding on for dear life with all my might

My body is tired, my body is weak
From you, God, peace for me I seek
The road is long, the battle rough
I no longer am strong and tough

I do not think I want to live this way
I question if I want to stay
Sometimes coming home to You
Is all I really want to do

But I will try and keep up the fight
Trying to make each day bright

HOLDING ON FOR DEAR LIFE

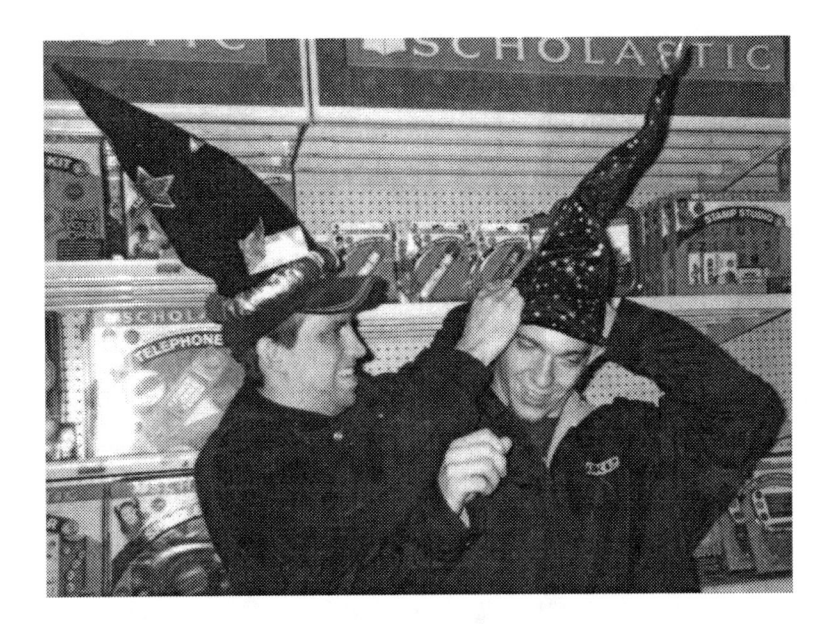

Chad and Shawn Having Fun in a Toy Store

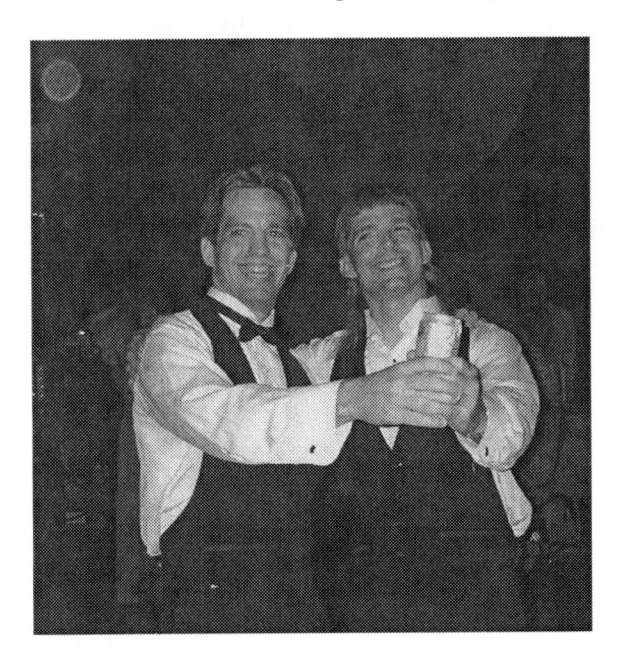

Chad and Joshua Having a Wedding Dance

The week to follow we started to see even more improvement. Chad was starting to feel better and becoming more talkative. The rash was going away and they changed his intravenous magnesium to oral pills. Again another medication that would have daily dosage changes depending on results of his daily lab work. He still continued taking the pain pill for his complaint of headaches and now right shoulder pain. After getting approval from the doctor I went to the store and got a heating pad for him to see if that would help relieve some of the discomfort. For whatever unforeseen reason his white count dropped as it did back when he was getting his chemotherapy and he needed a shot of Neupogen.

It was not until his clinic visit on day eighteen (December 30th) that we got results back from the biopsy they had done on the rash. It came back negative for GVHD. As Chad was able to sit out in the recliners more frequently now, he and Eric met and started becoming friends. Often they would look to see if the other was there upon arrival to the clinic and try to get recliners next to each other so they could visit.

Returning home from his clinic visit that day I received a phone call from the daily newspaper in my hometown in Kansas. They had heard of Chad's journey from a friend of mine. They wanted to know if they could do a story about Chad. We were surprised and thrilled. They interviewed Shawn, Chad and me. When I received copies of the article a week later it was very impressive.

That evening I placed a call to Shawn because it was his birthday and I did not want him feeling like I had forgotten or deserted him. I felt bad not being able to be with him as he was on his own. I felt bad that he was not able to be with us for Christmas. He reassured me that I was where I needed to be and that he was doing okay.

New Year's Eve was not celebrated by staying up to watch the New Year come in. We would be arising early the morning of New Year's day to go to the clinic for our regular early morning daily visit. Once again I thanked God for letting us have Chad there to see another year go by. I wrote a note on my calendar that said, "How can you protect someone from something you have no control over?" I look back at it now and it just seemed to confirm the helplessness I was feeling.

At our visit to the clinic, a sample of Chad's nasal secretions was taken. Even though the over the counter medication seemed to be helping he was still complaining of a stopped up nose, sneezing and having to blow his nose frequently. It would be a few days to get the test results back from the samples.

Chad had now progressed enough with his eating that he could eat an entire bowl of cereal and was not vomiting after each time he ate. The shoulder pain still was consistent and the heating pad did not seem to be giving any permanent relief. The Oxycodone was becoming a regular daily medication for pain. With this drug we had to get a new prescription written each time it was filled. It was a narcotic and habit forming.

The prescription had now run out and the doctor recommended he try using acetaminephen instead of the pain medication. This pain medication is one that a patient is supposed to be weaned off of but the doctor made him stop abruptly. It was a difficult time for Chad to be dealing with withdrawal symptoms. He was started on an antibiotic for infection, one pill five times a day for seven to ten days. The doctor also recommended moist heat to the shoulder followed by range of motion exercises. We inquired of having our family chiropractor see him for a possible adjustment to see if that would bring any relief. The doctor said it would not hurt anything but they really did not recommend chiropractors.

On day twenty-six (January 7th) Chad began complaining of blurred vision along with the continued shoulder pain. I asked of the use of a topical muscle medication and was approved to try it. An x-ray was taken of the shoulder but no problems could be found. The Prograf pump was discontinued and Chad was started on oral Prograf medication and Loperamide. It was explained to us that the blurred vision was a side effect of the medication.

Returning back to the house after Chad's visit he proceeded to the back door as he always did. He started up the back steps to the sun porch that led into the kitchen. There were about eight brick steps that he had to go up to get to the landing to enter the back door through the sun porch. On his ascent about halfway up the steps his foot slipped and he fell. I was horrified. I dropped the medication bag and my purse and ran to his side. I helped him to get up and looked him over. He had a few scrapes but no blood. After settling him into the house and checking him over more thoroughly we cleaned up the scraped areas and applied ointment and bandage. I knew we would need to watch for any bruising that could still make itself known later. He was still taking the blood thinner medication.

Rachael then placed a call to the family chiropractor. The chiropractor was able to have Chad seen that afternoon. Rachael took him to the chiropractor who made the adjustments that were needed and returning home Chad rested. He stated that he did feel less pain.

For the next fifteen days the biggest problem seemed to be that the level of nausea and vomiting had increased and Chad was frequently placed in the room at the clinic that had a bed where he could lie down.

At times, upon our arrival to the clinic, I would have to get a wheelchair to take him up to the fourth floor where the clinic was located. He would be too weak and ill to make the walk. Upon entering the clinic they would place him to bed and give him a shot to try and help relieve the nausea and stop the vomiting. Two or three times a day Chad was requiring oral doses of medication to get relief from his side effects of some of the medications and from the transplant.

Prograf levels were taken routinely to monitor the level amount and what it was doing to his body. If the level was not kept at a constant safe range it could cause serious side effects or even death.

During the daily blood work it was discovered that he was starting to get CMV viral infection. CMV is a very common virus that may or may not cause obvious illness in a healthy person. A portable intravenous pump with antibiotics was attached to the IV port in Chad's chest. A diet high in protein was recommended and we were to add peanut butter, marbled meats, pasta with olive oil, macaroni with cheese and ice cream to his diet and use half & half milk instead of whole milk and for him to drink only purified water. For some time we had been giving Chad purified water to drink as that had been recommended from the beginning with chemotherapy. We also added a drink with electrolytes. That visit he still continued to voice about the shoulder pain.

On day thirty-four (January 15th) the IV catheter in Chad's chest would not work and they had to work with it to get it opened back up. He was still taking the blood thinner medication but there was some problem with the port itself evidently. From that day on they had difficulty with it quite frequently.

It was recommended to add a nutrition drink to Chad's diet. We tried several different brands but none of them were acceptable by Chad. We finally gave up and concentrated on foods and other drinks such as the drink with electrolytes and juices.

Diarrhea and constipation were becoming a problem now. Sometimes we would have to give him anti-diarrhea medications and other times laxatives. It seemed to Chad that there was no relief from one symptom being taken care of to having another one start. Never did he voice his aggravation or disgust in putting up with all this turmoil.

On day thirty-nine (January 20th) Chad ate his first full meal since transplant and did not vomit. He also rested well that night. It was a milestone and a step towards renewed hope that the nausea, or at least the vomiting, would finally be stopping.

By day forty-two (January 23rd) Chad's appointments were finally changed to afternoons from mornings. That was a most welcome sound to Chad's ears. He would be able to sleep in and get the much-needed rest his body was craving for. I welcomed the opportunity to stay out of the morning rush hour traffic. A test was done to check on the viral infection. The results came back negative, meaning that the infection was gone. The IV antibiotic was done so the portable pump was removed, freeing him to move about without taking it with him. Chad's spirits were on the rise and he was in good humor.

Another milestone came on day forty-three (January 24th). We were informed that he was doing well enough that we could start coming to the clinic every other day. The doctors had become concerned about Chad's frame of mind and lack of rest and thought it best. I think they were also becoming more and more concerned that he had not gotten any signs of GVHD and wanted him to be able to be at home as much as possible. A welcome break from daily clinic visits and drives in Atlanta traffic also brought with it the concern that no GVHD could mean certain death in the near future for Chad.

The following appointment Chad had to return home with another portable IV pump because his magnesium level was dropping. With this medication I could discontinue the pump once the dose was in so it was not constant as were the other times with the IV pump. Chad said he knew how women felt carrying a purse around all the time. He frequently would wake from a nap and forget that it was there until he started to walk away and it would pull a little.

Over the days there were still times of loose bowel movements and changes in his magnesium and potassium levels that were addressed with changes to the medication regimen. The nausea continued but the vomiting became less and less. Chad's appetite began to increase to where he was able to eat larger portions of food.

During our clinic visit on day fifty-six (February 6th) Chad mentioned to the doctor that he thought his ADD (attention deficit disorder) was returning. When Chad was in middle school he was diagnosed with ADD. During his high school years he was on medication but that was stopped after he got out of high school. This was addressed by the doctor by increasing his antidepressant drug he was already on.

Over the next week Chad complained of feeling like he was getting a cold, feeling blah, having a sore throat and becoming shakier in his movements. He was sleeping frequently as he felt weak and tired after short times of activity. It was decided by the doctor that this was caused by the increase in antidepressant. The doctor changed his antidepressant to another brand.

Chad was gradually feeling a little stronger with each week that passed so Rachael ordered a treadmill for him to use in the house. He also began taking short walks outside with hesitation for fear of getting bitten by an insect again. Slowly his strength started improving.

Chapter 17
February 2003

Hopes of a New Day

There is now hopes for a new day
It looks as if this mountain is going away
The sun now shines brighter as time passes by
There is new hope that I may not die

A long hard fight may now be won
I can consider now having some fun
Away from the conflict and back into life
Enjoying things, me and my wife

Looking ahead to new goals made
As memories of illness now fade
Happiness now comes with simple things
As new life time now brings

Over the course of the past two months, Chad was not the only one that was getting routine medical care. Rachael had started her tedious regimen to prepare for an in vitro pregnancy. There were numerous shots, tests and visits that she had to schedule around her busy work schedule.

On February thirteenth Chad and Rachael went to the in vitro clinic so that she could have her ovarian eggs distracted. The eggs from Rachael were then paired up with the sperm from Chad that he had banked. Another clinic visit for her followed three days later. Chad and Rachael went to the clinic to have the fertile eggs placed inside her uterus. Now we had to wait until her following visit to see if they stayed intact.

I thought about how I used to think it was messing with God's plan for nature to have eggs and sperm reproduce in a test tube. God opened my eyes and my mind to the miracles He has taught man to perform. For without this process Chad would have never gotten to be a father and, lest I forget, me a grandmother.

On day seventy-two and seventy-three (February 22nd and 23rd) Chad felt well enough to go out and about with Rachael. Upon returning from their little trips he would feel tired and have some nausea but it was a good mental boost for him to be out amongst life again. He was always excited when he and Rachael could get out of the house and spend some time together. On returning to the house he was always cheerful and anxious to tell me of his adventure even though he would be tired and often nauseous.

Chad's birthday had arrived on February 25th. Rachael took Chad to his clinic visit that morning. During his clinic visit the new antidepressant was increased from once a day to twice a day.

I had gone to the grocery store to pick up items for the evening meal and to make a birthday cake. Upon returning I found Rachael and Chad back home and standing in the kitchen waiting for me. I could tell by the look on their faces that something was going on that I needed to be told. The news that hit my ears once again brought tears to my eyes. A home pregnancy test revealed that I was going to be a grandmother by the end of the year. For once, over the past two years, my tears were tears of much joy instead of sadness. The following week the home test results were confirmed at her doctor's visit.

To celebrate Chad's birthday he wanted to go to his favorite barbeque restaurant. He ordered the "all the ribs you can eat" dinner and went through three plates of ribs. You could tell he was enjoying every bite. Upon returning home he became nauseated and vomited but said it was worth every bite of it.

For the next three days he battled diarrhea but it was gotten under control. It was also recommended by his doctor that he try and avoid spicy foods.

A week and a half into taking the new antidepressant a personality change was noted in Chad. He became very short tempered to the point of being verbally mean. He seemed restless and was not sleeping well. During his next visit the new antidepressant was decreased back to once a day. The last treatment for his respiratory antibiotic was finished during this time. He was also given the okay to go to the dentist to get a tooth crowned that was much needed. It was something that had been delayed for several months for the fear of Chad having excess bleeding or getting infection.

I received a call from my younger brother's wife, Kelly, that the company she worked for was sending her to Atlanta for a training class. It was exciting knowing someone from the family was coming that we would get to visit with. Chad loved family and was thrilled that someone was going to be there to visit. We spent what time Kelly had available for a most wonderful visit. Chad was able to go out in public by this time so we ate at a restaurant. That was a joy to him to be able to eat a meal out. All too soon she had to return back to Kansas.

On day ninety (March 12th) we left the house to go for Chad's clinic visit. Upon departing we noticed traffic was very congested. We turned on the car radio to find out that there had been a semi-truck accident on the exit we needed to take to get onto Interstate 75. I proceeded down a side road. We had only gone about three blocks over a twenty-minute time frame. I contacted the clinic and it was agreed upon that we would change the appointment to the following day since Chad was doing well. Chad was so happy to hear that he got another day off from the clinic that he started singing to the music on the radio.

The following day we had no difficulty making his appointment. He still seemed irritable but was sleeping much better again. The irritation from the antidepressant was subsiding and his attitude was more positive. Elation came to Chad's entire outlook when we were informed that since he was doing so well he would now get to have three days off between clinic visits.

That next day there were times of nausea but very little vomiting. There were still the good days and the bad days but the good days were now finally outnumbering the bad ones.

After a second visit to the chiropractor most of the shoulder pain seemed to be relieved. The numbness in the hand was also easing up and going away. Outings other than to the clinic, however short, were set up for several times a week; that was a good mood booster.

Chad was starting to feel like he was going to survive and once again become a part of society. In the back of my mind lingered the fact that he was scheduled for another bone marrow biopsy on day ninety-nine (March 21st) and that would let us know if he were on the uphill climb to life or the downhill slide to death. He had still not gotten GVHD and that still concerned the doctors.

Chapter 18
March 2003

Life's Decisions

In life there are many crossroads
Some will make you carry heavy loads
Some will be an easy step
Some will wear you out or give you pep

The road you choose is not always up to you
It may be something that you have to do
It is not always easy to make up your mind
What is best for you is what you must find

At times only one road makes any sense
Even if it is covered with hard times so dense
Lift your eyes and pray for the best
Sometimes you cannot just stay safe in your nest

Day ninety-nine from the date of transplant finally arrived. Chad had been up since four in the morning with anxiety and worry of the biopsy and the possible results. We departed early that morning for the clinic for the bone marrow biopsy to be done. Before we left Chad removed the boulder from his poster board.

When we arrived at the clinic the IV fluids were started and lab work done. He was placed in a room on a gurney and given partial sedation. I stayed in the room but could not watch the procedure. I had seen him go through too much pain already to watch him going through more. I was assured that even though he verbally complained of pain that he would not remember it.

As I worked on tying a quilt blanket that I was making for my upcoming grandchild, I listened to the conversation. The physician's assistant and nurses had been talking with me about my manuscript I was working on as Chad was being given his unconscious sedation. While the procedure was going on he was telling them that he was going to have me put in this book that the nurses were mean and that the physician's assistant was the meanest of them all. We all laughed. We knew he was joking because he spoke very highly of the staff at the bone marrow clinic. Even during times of unconscious sedation he found humor. Occasionally Chad would let out a verbal statement that the procedure hurt. They reassured me that he would not remember any of it.

Once Chad was awake and recovered from the biopsy we went back to the house for him to rest. The stress and worry was getting to both of us and he was relieved that the procedure was over with. Now we all had to wait on the results and prayed.

The winters in the south are mild with seldom a fall of snow and spring weather comes in March. The days were comfortably warm with the mornings and the evenings still a little cool. We had decided it was perfect weather and timing to go on a short road trip to the mountains. Chad welcomed the idea with open arms. It had been a long time since he had taken a trip or gotten out of Atlanta. His trips in the past were something that he always loved. It had been a very long winter and we all three needed a break. After getting approval from the doctors, I reserved a motel room in Helen, Georgia.

It was about a two-hour drive from Atlanta, not too far if Chad had problems, but far enough away from the hospital to make me anxious if something did go wrong. Rachael and I packed that evening before departure as Chad rested.

The following morning, before leaving the house, Chad removed the last stone of one hundred days from the mountain I had made him with the poster board. Once all boulders and stones were removed the picture of the sun and the rainbow with the words "U R OUR HERO" were revealed. He smiled with pride that he had lived to remove that last boulder. He had taken that long road with all its pains and emotional stress and survived it all.

It was a peaceful drive going on winding roads looking at the tree-covered mountains. The stream we saw looked so crisp, clear and cool as it ran along the side of the road. Once in Helen we checked into our motel room and went out about the town to see what it was like.

A restful night's sleep brought new adventures the following day. We panned for gold and actually found some. We panned for gems and got some of those also. We shopped the quaint interesting little stores. I found three little bell angels with the names of Chad, Shawn and Rachael on them. They now sit out for me to look at every day to remember the fun, love and laughter we shared during that trip. I often think of the movie I had seen several times where it was spoken of how when you hear a bell ring it means an angel gets his/her wings.

That evening we returned back to Atlanta. After returning, Chad had four days of rest before he had to return back to the clinic for his next visit. On examination at his visit it was discovered that he had another viral infection and cold sores in his mouth. He was started on antibiotics once again.

The day after our return I placed a call to Eric's wife. Chad and Eric had become good friends since December 12th, their mutual date of transplant. Chad and Eric's clinic visits did not always fall on the same day. To keep in touch they occasionally called each other to talk and would select reclining chairs next to each other at the clinic to visit when they were there on the same days.

A date was set to meet them at a restaurant for the "100 Day Celebration." We all had a wonderful visit and enjoyed a fine meal. Before the night was done Eric and Chad decided that, as soon as they could, they would sit out on a porch together and have a beer while Chad taught Eric how to play guitar. Alcoholic beverages, of course, had not been any part of their diet for some time. Often they spoke of the beer on the porch when they visited.

Chad had played guitar ever since I bought him one and taught him how to play chords when he was in about the fourth grade. Over the years he taught himself how to play notes and got help from others on progressing his playing skills. Chad was building himself a collection of special guitars that he was very proud of. He had become a very good guitar player, though he never gave himself the credit he deserved. Eric had always wanted to learn how to play guitar and so Chad and he had plans for Chad to start teaching him. A strong friendship had bonded.

Two weeks had passed since we had seen Eric at the clinic. We figured he was getting more frequent days off now also and his clinic visits were no longer coordinating with Chad's visits. On occasion Chad would place a call to Eric but only received his voice message.

The following week at Chad's appointment I questioned one of the clinic nurses of his whereabouts. I was informed that he had been admitted to the hospital and was in the Intensive Care Unit and that he had gotten pneumonia. To my dismay I went to the ICU family room to find his wife, mother, father and sister. We hugged and I told them that prayers and thoughts would be with them.

It was not easy telling Chad about where Eric was and the condition he was in. My heart was heavy as I told Chad of the news. Our hearts ached for Eric and his family. As like Chad, Eric had great hopes of recovery, of him and his wife starting a family and of him and Chad sharing a beer on the porch.

Three days later at Chad's next scheduled appointment, I had plans to inquire of Eric's condition and to visit again with his family. Before I could ask, one of the nurses took me aside and informed me that Eric had passed away. I went outside and wept. Once I got control of my emotions I proceeded back inside to tell Chad of the sad news. It was difficult for him, as well was expected. That type of event was a harsh reminder that he was not "out of the woods" yet. On top of that he had now lost a good friend. We did receive some much-needed good news to offset the bad that day. Chad's bone marrow biopsy had come back clean.

Chad's visits were now going to be changed to weekly trips to the clinic. He was starting to eat better and gain weight. He was starting to have more energy as each week passed. His outlook on life was improving.

Occasionally he would still have to get a bag of IV fluids with his visits but this was an improvement from the two to four bags that he would get in the past. His medications were still monitored and changed as needed by his lab work results. Some of the medications were now discontinued as Chad progressed to improvement.

April was not only bringing in showers but new hope for the future. It was time for me to return back to Kansas. The doctor had given approval for Chad to be alone for short periods of time while Rachael was at work. The thought of leaving was difficult. This had so much become like home to me and I had made good friends and acquaintances.

Part of my reluctance to leave came from fear. I continued to carry the fear with me that Chad may not get the GVHD and things would turn for the worse again. I did, however, know that, for newlyweds, it was time for the mother/mother-in-law to leave. I knew in my heart that Rachael was glad and relieved that I was there to help with Chad and around the house while he was ill. But now that he was feeling better they needed to have their married life back and I was not needed for that.

Chapter 19

To Chad with Love

I have a son so warm and sweet
His birth was such a joy
Your big blue eyes swept me off my feet
That feeling of a first born baby boy

Your hair was soft brown at first
Then a touch of Great-Grandpa's red
Then turned blonde with sunlight's burst
On the pillow where you lay your head

Your eyes are big and blue and bright
Your heart is warm with love
You marvel at all things in sight
From deep at sea to the sky above

Your two little hands search all things
Your tender feet can be swift
You like to laugh and play and sing
To me you are truly God's gift

I had Tina and Shawn fly out to Atlanta so that I would not have to make the long drive by myself and to support my emotional departure. Shawn stayed with Chad in Atlanta and Tina and I took a quick trip to the coast.

While in Savannah/Tybee Island I voiced to Tina that Georgia had started to feel like home and I felt like my heart belonged in Savannah. At the time I had not realized that with each visit to Savannah its culture and beauty filled my veins more and more. I did not realize that I was planting the seed of an idea that would grow with much strength. A peacefulness was found inside me in the surrounding of the historical district and the beach. When on the beach I felt I was closer to God there than anywhere else in the world for Him and me to have our talks. I wondered if this was the same effect this city was having on Chad that drew him to it so strongly. I now knew what he had been trying to describe to me.

On our return to Atlanta I packed my belongings and my almost-two-year-old cat Whiskers and the four of us were headed down the road. I had gotten Whiskers at the age of nine weeks. He was born on Good Friday and I picked him up on the weekend of Mother's Day. He had become a good traveler and comforting companion for me both on and off the road. He adjusted well with all the changes from one home to another and the car traveling.

Shawn had just turned twenty-one and wanted to try his hand in a casino. We stopped in Metropolis, Illinois, to take a break from the drive and for his first experience with gambling. I had told him to play a certain slot machine. He did not want to leave the one he was on so I sat down at it. You can imagine the expression and disbelief on his face when I got a nice payout after the second or third pull. He decided after that that he would heed my hints. I divided out my little winnings between the three of us to continue playing. In just about thirty minutes or less we were all three tapped out and ready to continue our journey to Kansas. I did save some back to help deter the cost of the return trip.

We left Tina at Joshua and Melissa's home and Shawn and I continued our drive back home. Shawn was now living in the apartment with his girlfriend Cathy. Since my great uncle Archie had been asking me frequently to move in with him, I obliged. He was in his eighties and living alone. We had lost Great Aunt Alice, his wife, only a few years before at Easter time. He was glad to have the company and the help. It was nice to remove some of my belongings from storage and have them out again. I returned to work and on the surface all things seemed to be getting back to normal. On the inside I was dealing with much turmoil.

I tried to keep busy with work and cleaning and painting inside Great Uncle Archie's home. Kansas just seemed like a strange place now. I was there physically, all but my heart and mind. It was nice to be closer to family but difficult being farther apart from Chad. Knowing that my first grandchild was going to be living that distance from me also sat on my mind.

When I would talk to Chad and Rachael the reports were that Chad was continually progressing slowly. He was getting to enjoy events in life again. All seemed to be going well for him and Rachael. I did not want to interfere with their lives but the battle in my mind was overpowering. I kept having flashbacks of the times when I feared Chad's death when he was so very ill. I feared that I would receive another phone call, as I had when all this began. I worried that Chad would be alone if he received any bad news if he went out of remission. It would be like him to take himself to an appointment if he felt up to it.

Yet I had Shawn there in Kansas. I felt that I had all but deserted him during all this time and felt I needed to be there for him. Guilt was playing me from both sides. I prayed for God to lead me in what I should do.

One morning I awoke and knew my decision and stood firm to it. My decision put all my family and friends in awe and disbelief. No one could believe I was leaving a good government job and just up and moving to a place where I knew no one and did not even have a place to live or a job waiting. I was moving myself halfway across the United States with not a clue what was waiting for me or what I would encounter. My heart and determination were overriding my mind, they said. Chad and Rachael were thrilled with my news.

I felt that God was behind my decision and determination. I wanted to have both my sons close by me again. There were only four of us in our little family and I wanted us all close again as we had been when the boys were younger. We had family member number five to be arriving soon also. Besides, I was tired of the cold, snowy winters and constant wind on the Kansas plains. My younger sister's only comment summed up everyone's thoughts, "We should have figured that you would move to live by a beach someday the way you like the ocean and beaches." Her words rang true but my love for my little family was the final decision maker.

That morning in May I prepared for work as I always had. Upon arriving at work I went to see my boss. I truly do not think that he was totally surprised when I announced to him that I was giving a two-week notice and moving to Georgia. My co-workers offered to dump sand in my backyard and buy me a pool if I would stay. I refused the offer. They then said that they would also take shifts running by flapping their arms and making seagull sounds too as they played a tape of ocean wave sounds. I told them I would miss them and would keep in touch but was still going.

After work that day I went over to see Shawn and informed him of my decision and make him an offer. I wanted to know if he wanted to make the move with me. He said he did but wanted to bring his girlfriend with us. I informed him that if he wanted to make such an offer to her to make the move he would have to take her as a fiancé or as a wife. I was not paying for gas, motel, food, room and board for a girlfriend. His response to me was to ask me if I would go with him to help him select a wedding ring set.

Next I broke the news to Great Uncle Archie. He was not happy about me leaving but totally understood. Several times he stated that he would be out and visit whenever he could. I told him I would be happy for him to come stay.

When Shawn made his decision to move with me he traded his car for a pickup truck that needed a new engine. In two days he had it ready to go. Funds had gotten down to very little and I could not afford a moving truck for that long of a haul. Great Uncle Archie helped me to find a flatbed trailer and Shawn had some of his friends help build a large wooden box on it. It was not the prettiest sight but served the purpose well.

We had a farewell barbeque in my great uncle's backyard. That is where Shawn made his proposal. Shawn got down on one knee and proposed with a ring that was the cheapest and ugliest we could find. Cathy did not hesitate to say "yes." He then pulled out the wedding set that he had asked me to help him select. I knew that if she would accept his proposal with that awful ring then she would most likely stand beside him through thick and thin.

The next few days were spent packing, having a garage sale and saying goodbye to family and friends. They were sad goodbyes yet happy goodbyes. The idea of being farther from family but now having my own family together again warmed my heart. We could not risk Chad moving away from his doctors in Atlanta and I do not think moving back to the Midwest was in his heart.

Chapter 20
May 2003

Follow Your Heart

Time seems to go faster as you age
And you feel you have lived your life in a cage
Where you are is no longer where you want to be
From this trial in life you want to flee

You want to venture to a different shore
Or walk towards a new open door
Your life you want to move forward on
But all too quickly life chances are gone

If your heart tells you it wants to move ahead
But you are too weak to move from your bed
Just think of what you will regret
When it is too late and your maker you've met
Then the chances are gone

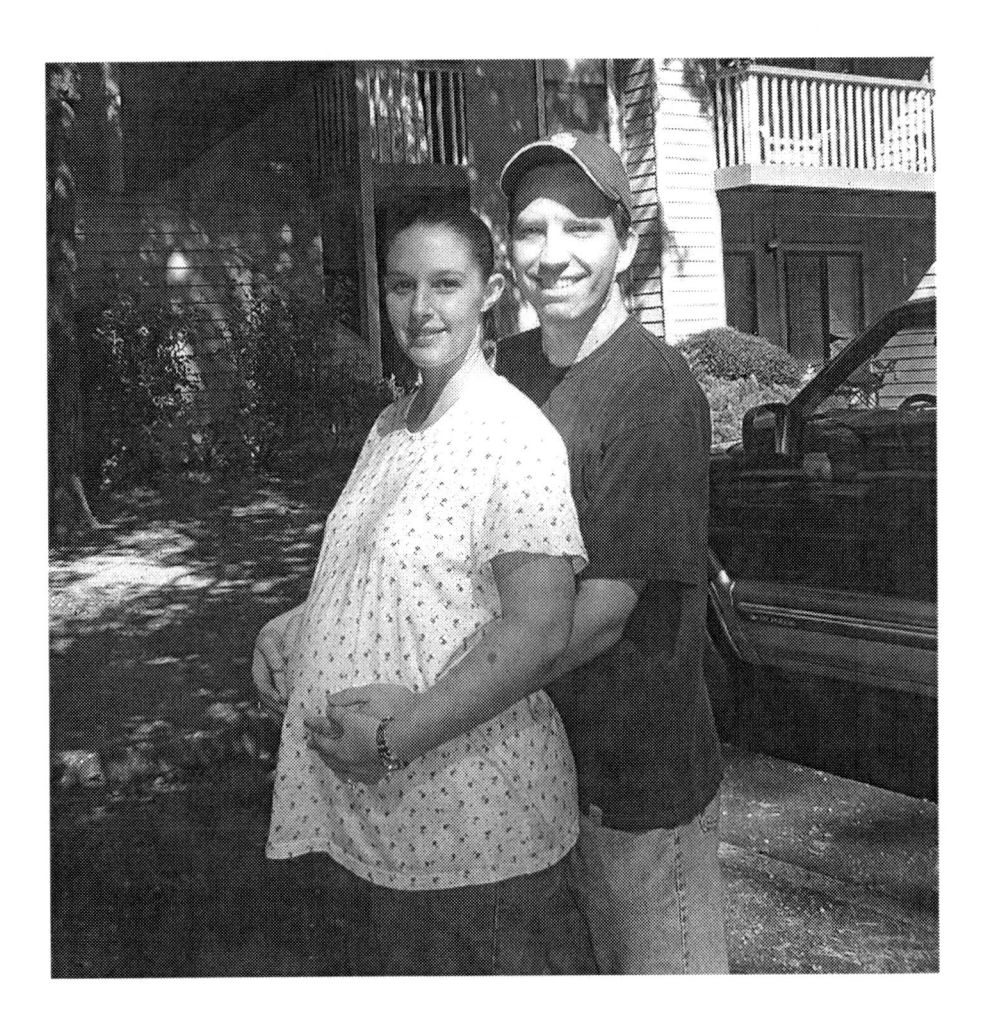

Awaiting a Special Gift

The day to move from Kansas to Georgia had finally arrived. It was May 25th. I was excited to get on the road. I had never pulled a trailer before so it was going to be a new experience. I was looking towards the move as an adventure. We were to make a stop at Chad and Rachael's in Atlanta where I would leave the trailer until I got a place in Savannah to live.

The time of departure arrived and we were off down the highway like a caravan. I led, pulling the trailer, Shawn was in his pickup behind me and Cathy followed in her Jeep. Shawn and I had cellular phones and Shawn and Cathy had walkie talkies that I had gotten for the trip. I knew it was going to be important to be able to keep contact between all of us while on the road.

We had gotten about twenty miles down the interstate and all seemed to be going well. As I was passing under a bridge a semi truck sped by me causing the trailer to jackknife back and forth. I prayed as I could see the trailer sideways in one side view mirror and then the other going from side to side. Once I got it corrected Shawn was calling me on my cell phone telling me to pull over and he would drive my SUV and pull the trailer. I thought of how when you fall off a bicycle you get back on. I told him I would stop at the rest stop ten miles down the road. I wondered if this was a sign that I was making a mistake. Still the inner push came to keep moving forward.

At the rest stop we unloaded and reloaded the trailer to distribute the weight better. For some reason we did not have the space we had when we packed it the first time so we had to leave a few items behind in the park's dumpster. Two hours later we were back on the road again heading east. I drove slower and more cautiously the rest of the way. When there would be a semi truck coming up from behind me Shawn would call and tell me so I would be prepared for the gust of wind that it would bring. The drive through the mountains north of Chattanooga and the traffic going into Atlanta had me nervous but I did well. Occasionally I began to doubt the decision I had made to make the move as each obstacle presented itself along the way.

It took two days to get to Atlanta. During those two days I questioned in my mind several times if I was doing the right thing. In my mind I knew I was moving to a city where I knew no one, had no job and did not even have a place ready to move into. I had accumulated large amounts on credit cards to make the previous trips to Georgia and help with living and food expense and some of the medical costs for Chad. In my heart I kept hearing that all would be well and just keep going forward towards the east coast. A feeling would come over me that would calm my anxiety and fears.

Reassurance that I was making the right move came when there was the most welcome sight of Chad and Rachael's home and their smiling faces.

Chad looked healthy and was feeling good. Both of them were very pleased about my decision to make the move.

The following day we left the trailer in Chad and Rachael's yard and all loaded into two vehicles. Chad and Rachael took their car as they would need to be returning for her to go to work before us other three were ready to return. We left to go to Hilton Head where we would stay in a motel for three days. I was determined that I should have a place found for us to live by then. I would spend most of my time looking for a place to live and also get to spend some quality time with my little family all together once again.

The search was ruthless. I had not imagined that rent around Savannah would be so high in the areas I wished to live. My first search took me to the historical district and my second took me to the islands. I recall vividly sitting at a little table in a restaurant on River Street drinking iced tea while searching through the newspaper for leads on apartments that I would be able to afford that would be in a safe area. It was becoming obvious that I would have to look elsewhere about the city to find what I thought I could afford. I prayed for God to help me. I had no idea where these places were. I had only been in the historical district and on the islands with any of my visits in the past.

I was again beginning to wonder if I should have stayed in Kansas. I had just moved three people to a new place with none of us having a job, very little money and discovering the cost of living in the historical district and on the islands to be beyond my means financially. But I also knew there was no way I was going to pull that trailer halfway across the United States again and this was the place my heart wanted me to be. I continued to hold on to the faith that the decision to move was led by the Lord.

On the third day Chad and Rachael had to return to Atlanta so she could return to work. Shawn, Cathy and I moved over to a motel on Tybee Island to continue the search for housing.

Early the morning of the fourth day of searching I arose feeling doubtful and concerned. At the housing cost I was finding I could not afford more than two months of bills for the three of us on what money I had left for us to live on. I got dressed and got a cup of coffee from the motel office area and headed out for a walk on the beach. I talked to God as I walked along watching the gulls and pelicans getting their morning catch from the ocean and listening to the crashing sounds of the waves. I marveled at the wondrous colors of the morning sky as the sun was awakening the earth. I asked God to give me a sign that I was doing the right thing.

Shortly after my prayer I looked down and saw part of a conch shell sticking out of the sand. I went to move it with my foot and it did not budge. Bending down and picking it up I discovered it was a full medium-sized conch shell. This was a treasure to my shell collection I had started several years ago from visits to various other beaches.

Tina and I used to take "girl only" trips to places with beaches until Chad became ill. I would always bring back some type of "sea treasure" for the boys along with a souvenir. I thought of all the other sea treasures I would find if I stayed here. It was a sign of hope for me. I remembered that I was not in this alone and that there would be three of us that could bring income into the household.

I asked God to lead me on that day to where I was to live and to please let it be a nice, clean, safe place at a price I could afford. I was pretty sure I would not be living where I had hoped to live in the historical district or preferably the islands but it would be where God wanted me to be. I would have to settle for what could be found in the appropriate price range and just needed to get something found quickly. The cost of the motel rooms was taking a bite out of my savings.

Our first stop that day, in the home search, was to a low-income apartment complex I had found in an apartment magazine that was located on Wilmington Island. They had nothing available but called over to another apartment complex to see if they were still running a move-in special. The manager of the apartments gave me directions and we were on our way. In the back of my mind I thought how we could not afford it but since he had already called them we may as well go look at it.

After looking at the apartment and talking with the assistant manager, I asked how much their move in special was. To my surprise we landed a two bedroom, two bath apartment with a fireplace for five-hundred forty-five dollars a month. I thanked God several times. Not only did He find me a nice, clean, safe place to live at a price I could afford but He did bless us well because to our delight we now were going to live on an island. I had always wanted to be an islander.

We returned to Atlanta to spend a day with Chad and Rachael before I once again hooked onto the trailer and was ready to make the final trip to our new home. With delight, Chad and Rachael said they would be down for a visit as soon as we were settled in.

Upon arriving to the island I missed the turn for the street to the apartments. I pulled into the next road to turn around and it happened to be the country club. It was an enormous, fancy clubhouse with perfect landscaping. I think we must have looked like hillbillies to these people that abruptly stopped their golf games to watch this strange sight go through the circle drive. After the little scenic tour we got turned around and to the apartment to settle in.

The summer of 2003 was a good summer. Shawn, Cathy and I looked for jobs and spent as much time at the beach as we could get in. We were learning the ways of beach living, things to know about the ocean, the southern way of life in Savannah and the joy of family togetherness again. Shawn and I did some ocean fishing for the first time. Shawn informed me that the fishing poles we had brought with us looked like toothpicks compared to the fishing poles we needed now. Our poles were used for lake fishing in Kansas and not large enough or sturdy enough for catching the sea creatures we hoped we would catch. A trip to the store solved that problem. Life was looking up.

Chad and Rachael came down to visit several times. Chad would always look for sharks teeth but never seemed to find any along the beach. He always marveled at the waves and the treasures he would find and enjoyed finding little sea creatures to watch at night with a flashlight.

Raina came down to visit us with her young son, Caden, and Great Uncle Archie. Chad and Raina had bonded more as a brother and sister relationship than that of distant cousins over their younger years of growing up together. It was a joyful time as Chad and Rachael came to Savannah during their stay. It was heartwarming to watch as Chad spent time with four-year-old Caden. He taught him the ways of the ocean and how to boogie board. I thought to myself of what a wonderful father he was going to be. Chad loved all children. It was a great time that ended all too soon when our visitors had to return home.

That summer was a joy to see Chad once again enjoying life as he had before he had started his battle with leukemia. He was now in remission, gaining weight, eating well, had a return of energy and was his cheerful fun-loving self again.

Rachael's pregnancy seemed to be going well and our family would be adding a new member in the winter. I felt blessed in many ways. Since I lived in Georgia now, I got to be a part of seeing my granddaughter on ultrasound and hearing her heart beat before her birth. I got to relax and get rid of the stress that had overtaken me over the past few years. Chad continued to get stronger. Chad and Shawn were once again together enjoying each other's company.

Shawn was the first to find a job. Cathy and I still searched. As each month went by I became more worried of finances. The savings account was slowly depleting and I still had credit cards to pay off. Once again I was wondering if I had made the right decision to move. It appeared that financially I had made a bad decision but I was determined that I was not going back to Kansas for I felt Savannah was where I belonged and where God wanted me for now.

The assistant manager of the apartments and I were becoming good acquaintances as the days passed. Frequently I was at the office to fax resume's and sometimes just to visit with her. Our friendship grew as we talked more. Her words of encouragement during those times when my mind would tell me to tuck my tail and return to Kansas gave me strength and the will to keep pushing forward. Daniela would remind me of my strength and will to not give up.

Cathy got a job found working in a restaurant ocean side and I finally found a part-time job in a chiropractor's office. While working there I began making new friends and that gave me new hope that things were going to get better and be okay.

My world seemed to be wonderful and more perfect than it had ever been since before that dreaded phone call in Kansas when Chad's battle had begun.

Some friends and family were even telling me that they were envious of me and wished they had my life. I questioned that heavily as I knew what I had been through and the bills I was still facing. Not all things are as they appear. You must walk in the person's shoes to know their life. I have always tried to be a positive thinker and look to the good in everything. Perhaps that is what they were seeing.

All did seem like a perfect life until mid-July. Once again it was with the ringing of a phone that crashed my world.

Chapter 21
June 2003

A Soul Lost at Sea

I watched the tide come in today
It came from way out lost at sea
But in its rush it could not stay
It did not know where it should be
The waves pressed up against the sand
Then scattered, receding back to the sea
If it wanted to stay on the land
Why then did it flee
Upon the rocks it splashed and spewed
And fell between the jetty cracks
As if each droplet had been cued
To follow in each other's tracks
Yet there was a calm about the roar
And the rush upon the sand
As the waves came up the shore
To show its strength so grand
Our lives become confused as the tide
We lose and punish ourselves on the rocks
But as the receding of tears we cry
The door to a calm peace unlocks

Chad's visits to the clinic through the summer months continued but were spaced two to three weeks apart. In June he had another bone marrow biopsy done. We were told that there seemed to be some activity of the cells but not enough to be concerned about because it was still in normal range. Chad was beginning to put on weight as his eating habits returned to normal. He was feeling better and was once again able to get out among society and enjoy some of the events of normal life. He had stopped wearing only sweat suits and was now adorning himself in regular street clothes.

On one of my visits, he and Rachael took me to the Botanical Gardens. Chad loved being around all the plants and flowers. He loved nature and beautiful things that it would produce. As a child he had always marveled at seeing and doing new things. It was a peaceful place for him amongst the flowers, plants and little streams in all the turmoil he had overcome.

On July Fourth we all celebrated in Savannah. Chad mentioned that we broke the chance of a tradition by not celebrating at the hospital in Atlanta. We were all deeply and seriously thankful for that even though we laughed. I was thinking how I was glad we were not even in Atlanta the Fourth of July and wondered if Chad and Rachael were thinking the same.

We spent the biggest part of the day at the beach watching the speed boat races as they flew past us on the ocean waters. Chad noticed the television announcer for a sports television station and could not resist his antics. After getting our attention, he proceeded to waltz himself behind the announcer. Dancing past behind him he stopped long enough to give the peace sign by holding his first two fingers up in a V form. Most of all we just enjoying the fun of each other's company.

Chad dug down in the sand to make room for Rachael's stomach so she could tan her backside. She was well on her way to showing she was pregnant. He and Shawn spent memorable times riding waves on their boogie boards and skim boarding. We barbequed a lot and made wonderful memories. It seemed to be the perfect world.

Shortly after our July Fourth celebration I received the dreaded phone call. Chad had noticed a lump in his breast and had the doctor examine it. A needle biopsy was done to determine if it was cancer. There was a tumor in his right breast and one on the chest wall of the left breast. Once again fear reared its ugly head at us.

The needle biopsy confirmed that it was a tumor with cancer cells. The lump was surgically removed with hopes that they had gotten it all.

Due to the results of the biopsy, more studies and tests were ordered by the doctor. Chad had a CT scan done of his chest and abdomen. The lungs were clear but there were two stable cysts that were found in his liver. All other organs were found to be normal. A Doppler test was done on his right testicle and two small masses were found. Another bone marrow biopsy was done that came back clean. I was a little confused as to all these specific areas that were showing up to have cancer cells yet there were none found in his bloodstream as leukemia.

Due to theses finding and the fact that Chad had still not shown signs of getting GVHD gave much concern. The doctors began a new regimen of treatment on July 7th. Chad received an infusion of his bone marrow donor's lymphocytes and a dose of high-dose Ara-C chemotherapy for relapse. Electronic beam radiotherapy was given to the lump areas on his breasts. A lumbar puncture was done to test the spinal fluid and place chemotherapy medication into his spinal fluid.

On July 30th Chad received a second infusion of high-dose Ara-C chemotherapy that was followed by another infusion of his bone marrow donor's lymphocytes on August 13th.

The month that had started out as a celebration of independence was now ending with feelings of having nothing to celebrate. Once again Chad had lost his independence of quality of life to the controlling confines of cancer. In the blink of an eye his life would go from upbeat and positive to facing the fear of death at his doorstep once again. I made trips up to Atlanta to be with him as often as I could.

During the months of August and September Chad continued to go to the hospital for his spot radiation treatments to the masses in his testicle and for more frequent clinic visits. His outlook of life still seemed to be positive on the surface but deep inside was the ever wondering fear of if he were going to lose his life soon. He had spoken to Jeremy in the past and told him that he knew that he would never win this battle in the end and that his death was inevitable.

There were still no signs of GVHD evident so on September 19th he was given a third dose of chemotherapy and another injection of the first donor's lymphocytes.

Chad was now beginning to complain more of stomach discomfort. This brought hopes that there was some GVHD activity. Alas again it was not. Stress and worry was taking its toll on Chad's body now also. His hopes of winning the battle seemed to be in question in his mind. The stakes were higher now than before due to the fact that in two short months he was going to be blessed with becoming a daddy.

Another bone marrow biopsy was done on October 10th. The results came back again with some mild hypo cellular activity but we were told it was still in normal range, as it had been in June. According to the bone marrow biopsy, Chad was still in remission from leukemia.

Chad had now noticed a dark spot that had become evident on his leg. It was a small dark circle area that resembled the appearance of a dark bruise about the size of a dime. After an exam the doctor informed us that it was known as a curtis module and was a form of leukemia.

Six days later Chad was admitted to the hospital for another dose of chemotherapy followed by another dose of the donor's lymphocytes that had been stored for him. He was also infused with IL-2 that was to help in activation of the proliferation of T cells. This was in hopes to put the leukemia in remission again and to promote the possibility of Chad getting GVHD.

Chad had no specific complaints of pain but did feel weak and fatigued. Sores once again appeared in his mouth making it difficult for him to eat. Justifiably, depression started setting in and Chad began having a very serious outlook about everything. There was little laughter and very few words from him. It was as though he was closing himself in.

External beam radiation therapy was ordered for the dark spot on Chad's leg. He received twelve treatments over a five-day period to his leg and had received twelve treatments over a five-day period to the masses in his testicle. Chad tolerated these treatments well and spoke of how they were nothing compared to the total body radiation he had gone through previously.

The radiation treatments caused a decrease in his testosterone level. It dropped low enough that they thought they may have to do therapy replacement. They monitored the level and after one month it returned to normal levels so the replacement therapy was not needed.

Stress levels came down as it seemed the doctors were getting everything under control. Once again we were just waiting to see if Chad would get GVHD. Chad began to open up more but still carried some depression.

Chad came up with a name for himself since he did not have to have his other testicle removed. He now referred to himself as the uni-baller. This was a joke between him and Shawn. Once again it amazed me how he could find fun and laughter even with all he had been and was going through. Yet he took his own situation and found the humor in it.

Rachael continued to do well with her pregnancy and the expected date of arrival was any time. This was a very big incentive for Chad to do all he could to win this battle. We were all awaiting word from Rachael that she was ready to go to the hospital.

Chapter 22
November 2003

Miracle of Love

A baby girl conceived by love
A wonderful miracle from above
A gift of life for all the world to see
A part of you and a part of me

A flow of tears comes to my eyes
But it is in happiness that I cry
The joy and pride I see in you
Makes life worth fighting all I have been through

I hold your hand that is so small
I watch you as you learn to crawl
I look into your eyes of blue
I see my spirit inside of you

To hear you laugh warms my heart
Even though I know someday we will be apart
But I will be with you every day
As I watch you grow and play

Distance will not keep me away
By your side I will be, come what may
You are my sunshine and will always be
For you are forever a part of me

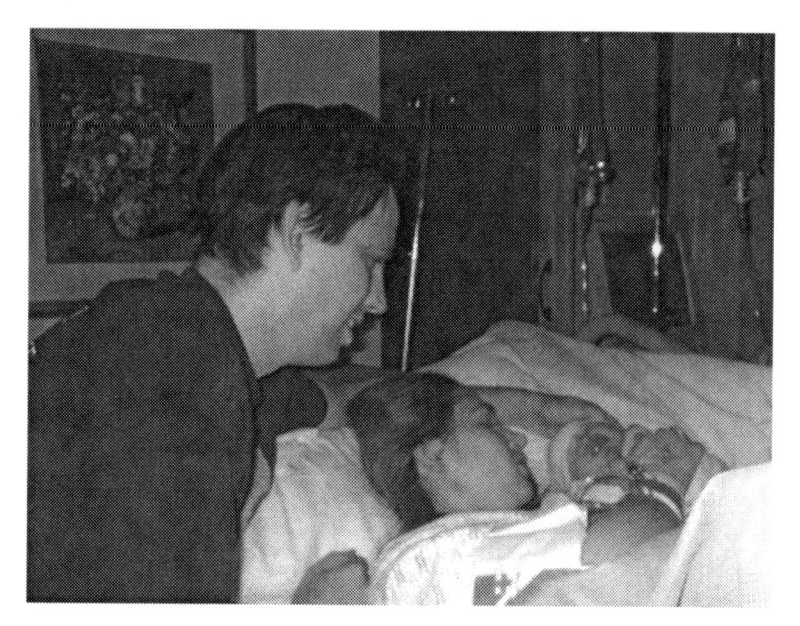

A New Addition to Our Family

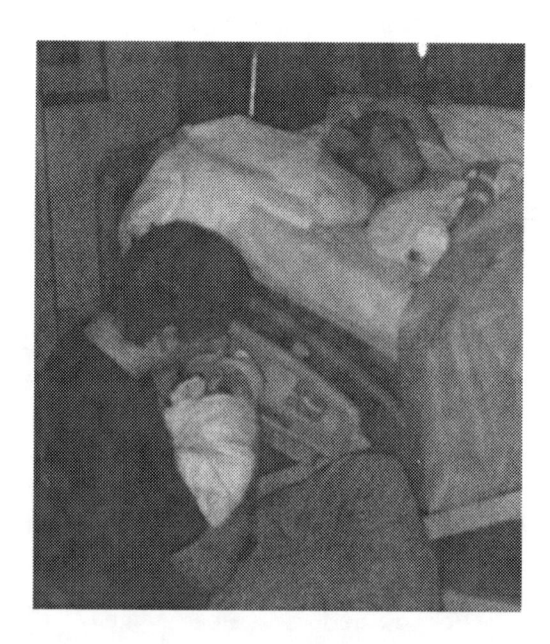

A Special Moment in Time

On the late afternoon of November 15th I received a phone call from Chad while at work. This time it was a most welcome phone call. Chad had taken Rachael to the hospital to give birth to our new family member.

I informed my boss and called Shawn to let him know and then I was out the door headed to Atlanta. I had packed a suitcase ahead of time that I had placed in the trunk just for this occasion. I prayed for God to let me make it to the hospital before Rachael had the baby. Somehow I made a four and a half hour trip into a three and a half hour trip. Only God knows how that happened because I did not drive any different than I usually would and I did not cross over a time zone.

I arrived at the hospital in plenty of time before the baby was born. The birth went well and mother and baby were both fine. Chad, Rachael's friend, and I were in the birthing room with Rachael, two nurses and the doctor. It was a moment like no other when we heard the first cry of new life.

The baby girl was placed in a bassinet in the room. She had ten fingers and ten toes. Very thick long dark brown hair and was a beautiful soft pink color.

I will never forget the moment that Chad and I stood, one on each side of the bassinet. We looked at this new little life and then at each other with tear-filled eyes and then hugged. We talked of how beautiful and perfect she was. We talked of how God had blessed us in the most wonderful way. The joy was overwhelming. Chad was beaming with pride and joy. I was so thankful that he was blessed to be alive to see and experience this very moment.

It was truly a miracle for our family to see this precious baby born into the world. If it had not been for Chad's first doctor telling us of using the sperm bank there would have been no way Chad would have ever been able to have a child. I thanked God for that doctor thinking to give Chad the insight along with so many other things I could think of at that moment to be thankful for.

Kiersten was dressed and wrapped in a little pink blanket and handed over to Rachael to hold. Chad stepped over to the bedside. Both parents looked overjoyed even though you could see the underlying signs of exhaustion on both their faces.

Soon it was Grandma's turn. Holding this child was like holding a piece of Heaven. She seemed so alert and attentive, watching my face intently as I spoke to her.

Kiersten did not want to sleep when she came into the world. Most of the first twenty-four hours of her life were spent awake. Of course being a new grandma I was more than willing to care for her so that Rachael and Chad could rest.

As her mommy and daddy slept I cuddled and rocked Kiersten. I held her out from me so we could look at each other. I told her how very special she was. It seemed as if we made a very special bond between the two of us during that time. As I talked and we looked into each other's eyes, she smiled at me.

Some say there is no way she would do that yet and others say she must have seen an angel or had gas. I know she smiled at me because I felt the moment we made our bonding connection in that split second.

During those first two days there was also a strong bonding made between Kiersten and Chad and Rachael. It was as though God had blessed her with a magical sense of being. It was as though she knew she was blessed with a family that would love her unconditionally to the end of time. She was so alert and seemed to have a sense of peace about her.

I had gone on to the house to prepare for the new family homecoming on the day of dismissal from the hospital. I wanted to make sure that the house was clean, the groceries gotten and all preparations ready for Daddy, Momma and baby. By late morning I heard the car pull up into the driveway. It was a proud and exciting moment when the family of three came in the door to start a new way of life together. A baby in the house was a blessing from Heaven that Chad and Rachael so much had deserved.

Kiersten's new life brought new life into Chad. He now had more reason to fight anything that would come his way in his battle. He talked of watching her grow and enjoyed every new thing that she would do. She was his sunshine. He would call me and talk with excitement in his voice with each new thing that his baby daughter would do. You could tell by watching him that he was still becoming fatigued easily but he was not going to let that rob him of this moment in his life.

As with anyone that has a new baby brought into the family, there were some major and some minor adjustments to make. In just a short time everyone seemed to be settling in to a more normal lifestyle. All things were getting into a new routine and Chad continued with his clinic visits.

On December 9th the doctors announced to us that since Chad had still not gotten GVHD and due to the areas that had presented themselves on his breasts, testicle and leg, they decided that it best to do another bone marrow transplant from a different donor. This was something that had rarely been done and would fall under the classification of research. However, when Chad was first given the options of chemotherapy or transplant during his initial diagnosis there was not that extra option as it was now.

Now through research he did have another chance, however slim it may be. There were no other choices to opt for to try and let that little girl have her daddy watch her grow. Once again the only other option was to do nothing, and that meant certain death in the near future. Bottom line was for Chad to let them try another bone marrow transplant donor or guaranteed death in his near future.

Again it seemed like all Chad had been through was in vain. Once again we were taken back to square one. However, this time they would not be able to do the total body radiation before the transplant. All the radiation that Chad received before his first transplant had taken his body as far too microwaved as it was safely possible. Any more total body radiation would start cooking his insides.

On that day the search began for finding someone to help save my son's life once again. He was placed on the portable IV pump with medication to assist with any GVHD that they hoped he may get. Depression set in severely again as he felt like he had come so many steps forward to only have to go back to the start.

Chad always looked forward to the Christmas holiday and loved decorating. One evening Rachael called me to tell me that Chad had insisted on placing lights on the eaves of their house. I was glad that she informed me of this little adventure of his after the fact! Chad had crawled up onto the roof with his portable IV, a hammer, hooks and lights and put the blue Christmas lights around the front and side of the house eaves. Determination has always been one of Chad's strengths and remained with him through his battle. His stubbornness, I must admit, I think comes from a little bit of a stubborn streak I tend to have. Once there is a mindset there is usually nothing that can be said or done to change the mind. I just thanked God for keeping him safe while he was doing this feat that he had no business doing.

Chad and Rachael had decided to spend Christmas in St. Louis, Missouri, with her family and have Kiersten baptized while they were there. This would be done by her father at the same church where their wedding had taken place.

Since they would be spending Christmas with her family, we set up arrangements to meet each other and do a gift exchange before their departure. We made plans to meet in Macon, Georgia, and have lunch and exchange gifts. After they returned from celebrating holidays in St. Louis they would come to visit me for our family Christmas get-together.

I had stayed in contact with my friend Monty over all these months. Once I had moved to Savannah Monty and I met each other in person for the first time. He always wanted to know how Chad was doing and awaited hearing of the birth of our new family member. I had called Monty to see if he would like to ride to Macon with me. This would give him a chance to finally meet three of the most important people in my life that he always heard me talk about. He was glad to ride along. I was thrilled to get to have him meet Chad, Rachael and of course our newest member to the family, Kiersten. He knew of who they were as we had been communicating over internet and then on the phone for over a year by this time. He was anxious to meet this brave, strong son that I had been speaking of and this beautiful new baby.

We all went out to eat lunch at a restaurant of Chad's choice. When the meal was finished and the bill came I reached for it. Monty grabbed it up and treated us all to our "Christmas dinner." A kind-hearted, Christian man was the way to describe him. He made the description proud for a true southern gentleman. He had been a rock for me to lean on and still continued to be just a phone call away when I needed to talk.

After our meal we exchanged gifts at our cars. From there we all went to the mall and walked and talked. It was a good time. I was so proud to be pushing Kiersten around in her stroller. We stopped at a little photo booth on the upper level that made black and white drawn pictures. With a little coaxing Chad and Rachael got their portrait done. Since Chad started this battle he did not like his picture taken. As the evening approached we said our goodbyes and went our separate ways.

On the way back to Savannah I thought of the Christmases that Shawn and I had missed out on. I hated that Chad and Rachael and Kiersten would not be with us but welcomed the thought that Shawn would be with me for this Christmas.

Christmas morning we opened our gifts. After eating our lunch we did something special that we had never before dreamed of doing on Christmas day. Shawn, Cathy and I went for a long walk on the beach. We all agreed that this was much better than the cold, and possible snow, we would have been walking through in Kansas. They both confirmed to me that this move was one of the best things that had happened in their lives.

When I left Chad, Rachael and Kiersten, I knew that that was the last time I would see them in 2003 and wondered what 2004 was going to bring Chad's way. And what it was going to bring to all the members of my little family.

As the year came to a close I sat and pondered about all that had been taking place over the past two and a half years. I also reminisced of past Christmases that I had experienced with Chad and Shawn.

On the evening of the last day of 2003 I wrote this poem to summarize my thoughts.

New Year Thoughts

Today is the last day of the year
Tonight you may celebrate with champagne or beer
But for now let us look at today
You do not want to throw the last day away

HOLDING ON FOR DEAR LIFE

Take time to count your blessings you got
Think of the battles you won and you fought
Look at the strength you found within you
To be brave and try something new

Take the time to look at those around you
Remembering friends, the old and the new
What part in your life did they play
Were they joyful or did they get in your way

During the year did you take the time to play
Did you stop to see nature's beauty on your way
Did you take time to count blessings you got
And thank God for winning the battles you fought

This is the end of two thousand and three
Nothing you do can stop its flee
Just prepare to tell it goodbye
And do not ask too many questions, "Why"

Today is the day to tie up loose ends
Perhaps it means calling a few friends
Do not let anything unsaid go out with the year
Or you may also lose a friend you hold dear

Look around at the things undone
Did you work too hard or have too much fun
There are probably a few things to complete
Do not start the New Year with too many irons in the heat

Look ahead to two thousand and four
With excitement as God opens each door
New adventures, new starts and newfound strength
Be brave, have faith and you will go the length
Make it a year to look on and say
"It was a great year, I did it God's way"

Chapter 23
January 2004

Silence of the Night

In the silence of the night
A pondering mind remembers the past fight
Unaware of the surrounding sounds
As the chains of leukemia bounds

Praying in the dark for another chance
To give life one more dance
To face the enemy in further fight
To try and make all things right

Once again a tear does fall by
As again you say "I do not want to die"
Courage and determination now build inside
As fear and pain you try to hide

HOLDING ON FOR DEAR LIFE

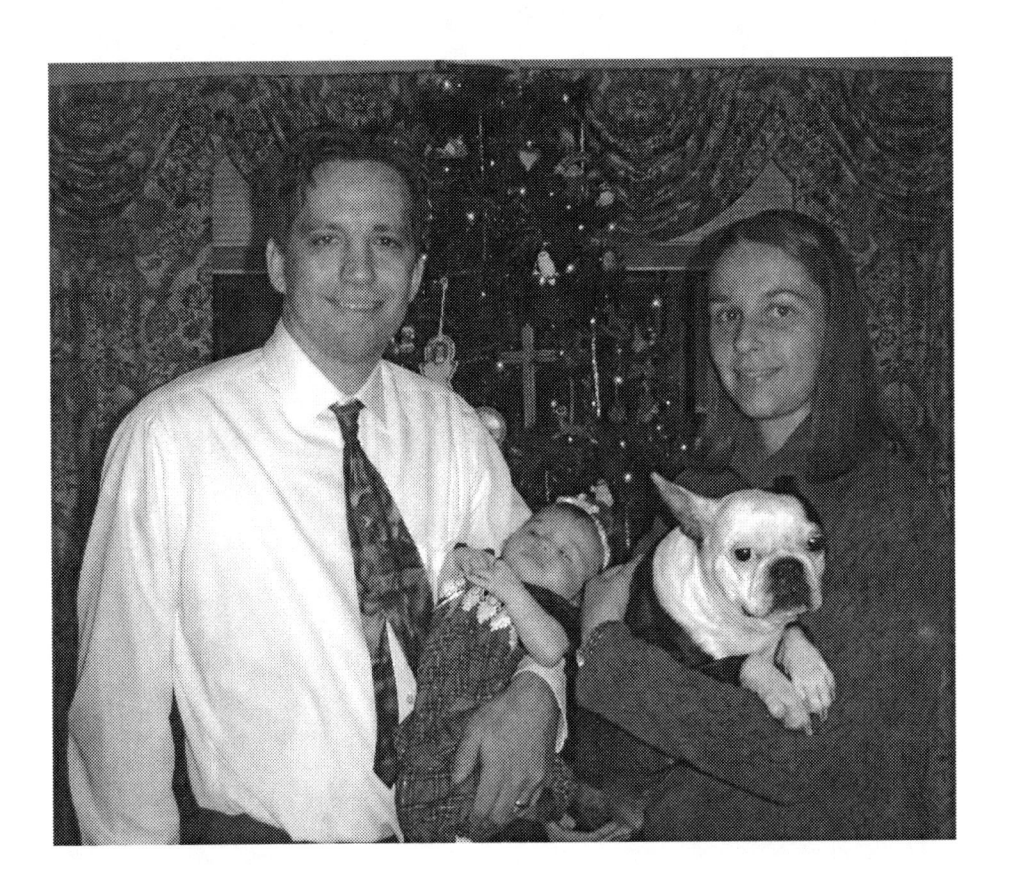

Kiersten's First and Only Family Christmas with Daddy

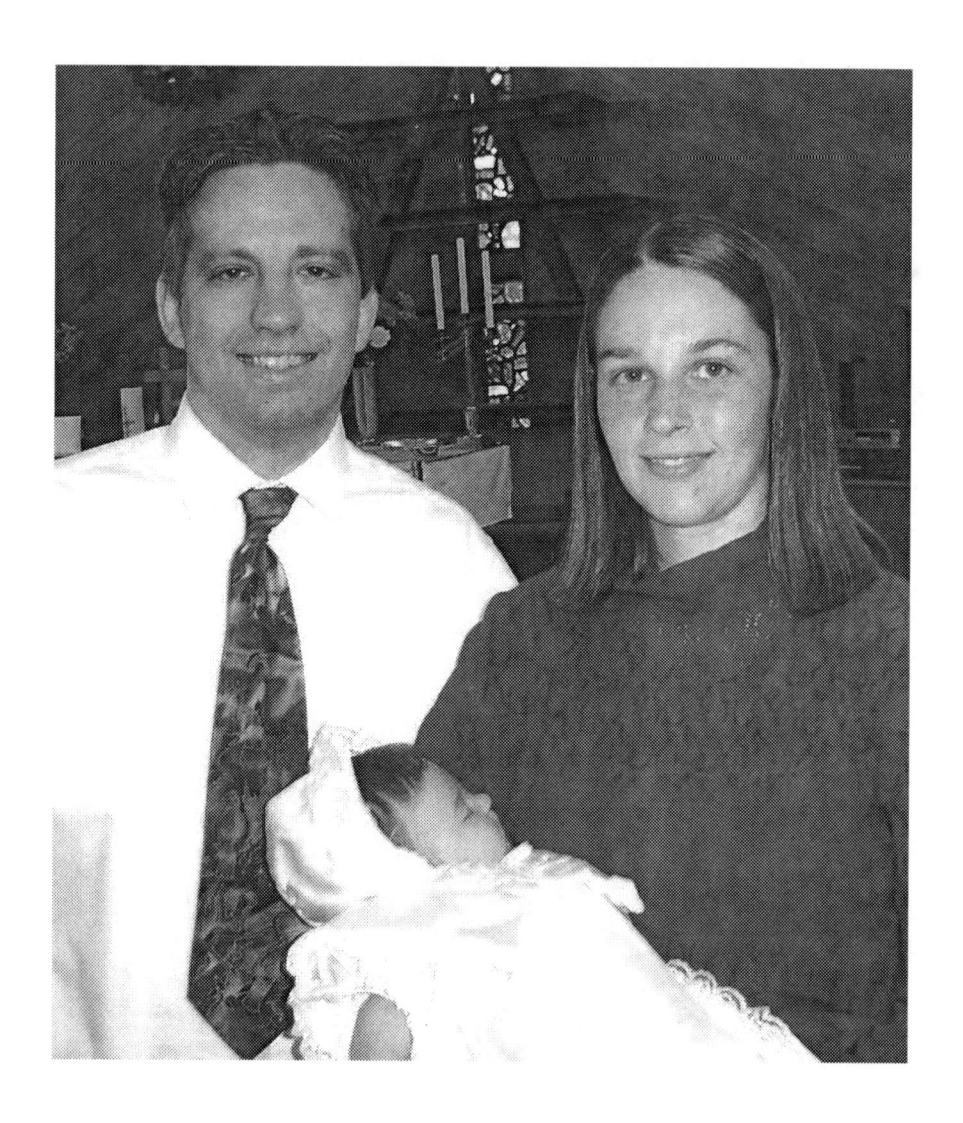

Kiersten Was Baptized in the Church
Where Her Mommy and Daddy Were Married

It had been difficult to find the first donor since Chad had a rare gene. We prayed and hoped for a new donor to be found. After the first two weeks of the search we were told that a donor had been found but that this person did not know for sure if they wanted to go through with the procedure to donate. Still preparations to do the transplant began for Chad.

Chad went through a battery of numerous tests that had to be done. He had been complaining of a cough and some fever so a chest x-ray was done first and results came back okay. The following day he had a pelvic and hip x-ray done that showed a mild contour weight-bearing irregularity in the right femoral head with a possible infarction. This meant that there was an area of necrosis in the tissue that was causing an obstruction of the local circulation by a blood clot. He was getting avascular necrosis. We were told that this was probably caused by all the radiation and chemotherapy he had received.

Avascular necrosis is a disease resulting from the temporary or permanent loss of the blood supply to the bones. Without blood, the bone tissue dies and causes the bone to collapse. The process involved the bones of Chad's hip joint; it could lead to collapse of the joint surface.

The evening after the first set of tests the doctor called to report that Chad had a pulmonary embolism that was discovered from the tests they had done. He was admitted to the hospital immediately once again. Chad was placed on bed rest and given shots to thin his blood.

A pulmonary embolism occurs when a blood clot breaks loose from the wall of a vein and travels to the lungs, blocking the pulmonary artery or one of its branches. This can block the blood flow from the heart.

A week later we received word again that the donor they had found was still reluctant and still had not decided if they would do the procedure for Chad to receive another bone marrow transplant.

A few days after Chad had been released from the hospital, Rachael called to let me know that the owner had sold the house they were living in. They were going to have to move. Chad would be unable to help with the move so it would be up to us. A call was placed to one of Chad's co-workers, a friend he had made when they had moved to Atlanta, Rachael's boss and her fiancé, and to her aunt and uncle who lived about an hour and a half outside of Atlanta.

We all met at Chad and Rachael's on moving day. I was placed in charge of caring for Kiersten and Chad. On the first move the couch went so that when we moved Chad he would have a place to lie down. While the others made the move I worked on emptying boxes and putting some items away while keeping an eye on Chad and Kiersten. The move went smoothly with the help that was given. Rachael was exhausted going back and forth between the houses and making sure that everything was done. Soon Chad's family was once again settled in at their new home about twenty minutes north of Atlanta. Once they were settled in I returned to Savannah.

This did not put a hold on the doctors preparing Chad for his second transplant. The next day at the clinic he was given his first high dose of chemotherapy to prepare for a peripheral blood stem cell transplant by a matched unrelated donor.

Two days later he received another dose of chemotherapy. With this clinic visit, Chad was placed again in the hospital for the blood clot and more chemotherapy. By this time Chad was doing everything he could to try and stay out of the hospital. It was the last place he wanted to be. He had spent all too much time around the hospital and clinics.

After three days the doctor said that they would let him do part of his preparatory medications at home as long as he followed the instructions to the letter. He could take the rest of his chemotherapy by pill instead of intravenously.

One evening he became very nauseous and was vomiting so much that he was unable to take his dose of chemotherapy medication. Instead of contacting the doctor that night he waited until the following morning at his clinic visit to let them know he had missed a dose. The doctor became very upset and put him into the hospital. We were informed that by missing that one dose it could interfere with the transplant severely. I went to Atlanta immediately.

During his first week in the hospital they did another bone marrow biopsy and a lumbar puncture. A CT scan of the abdomen that showed a new lump in the axillary lymph node, thrombosis (obstruction of an artery or vein by a blood clot) in the left lower lobe of the pulmonary artery, and a low density lesion in the left lobe of his liver. Next a CT scan of the head was done and that was okay except for the sinuses that showed inflammation and occlusions of both sinus cavities. The CT scan of his hips showed advancement of the avasular necrosis of both femoral heads of his hips with the right being affected more than the left and osteoarthritis setting in on the left hip with effusion and marrow edema and a tiny hyper-intense lesion in the left femur. The effusion was the escape of fluid from vessels by rupture that was causing the marrow swelling.

To follow all those tests was an echocardiogram that showed evidence of a mild mitral regurgitation in his heart with some pulmonary insufficiency.

This prompted a pulmonary function study of his lungs that showed decreased smaller lung volumes since the study that was done on November 2002. It also showed a possible emerging restrictive process, due to the possibility of development of parenchymal lung disease which would cause decreased lung volume due to an abnormal growth.

At the end of the intense week of tests an intravenous chest catheter was again surgically placed on the left upper side of Chad's chest. During this procedure they also did surgery to place a vena catheter filter. This filter is a tiny metal device that looks like an opened umbrella. It is inserted into the inferior vena cava (the large vein which returns the blood from the lower half of the body to the heart). The filter would catch blood clots that would originate in Chad's legs, or pelvis and keep them from advancing to the lungs, heart or head. I once again had fear running through my veins as I remained with Chad at his bedside.

Chad was exhausted and irritable by the end of the week and the following week brought no relief for him to rest either. Hip pain seemed to be increasing at a steady rate. He wanted to go home. Chad asked the doctor about letting him go home and to finish his preparatory treatments by clinic visit. The doctor that was on-call for Chad's regular doctor refused to dismiss him.

The doctor literally belittled Chad with his words of telling him how irresponsible and undependable he was. He also told him that, in his opinion, neither he nor Rachael was responsible enough to follow the medication regimen that had been set for him. I thought that to be a little out of line on the doctor's part as he carried it to the extreme. A mistake was made. I could not imagine that missing one dose from evening to morning could make that much difference.

Chad became furious and started to tell the doctor that since he had just been told that he will probably die anyway because he did not take that one medication dose at the scheduled time that he might as well go home to die.

The doctor was ruthlessly argumentative in talking with Chad, which upset him all the more. He told Chad that if he went home from the hospital on his own that they would no longer treat him. He reinforced that by missing his dosage of medication that the transplant probably would not work and he will die anyway.

Tears ran down his cheeks and he brushed his hand across his over-bed table making a can of soda fly across the room and hit the wall.

The doctor left the room and I tried to comfort Chad. He continued to cry and asking me to take him home. He had lost all hope about everything at hearing the doctor's words. He felt that if he had now ruined his chances of the second transplant saving his life he just wanted to be at home to die. In my anger I had a hard time figuring out why this doctor was so mean and hateful in his manner of conversation just over one pill that was missed. I felt furiously angry with this doctor for zapping all hope from Chad in just a few minutes that I had instilled over the past three years. I also knew that arguing with him at this point would only add to the aggravation and tension that had filled the room.

I told him that I would go talk to the doctor. After I regained my composure I told Chad I would be right back. I knew that lashing out at the doctor in anger or trying to argue with him would only make matters worse at this point.

I calmly approached the doctor in the hallway and he again reinforced that by Chad missing the medication the transplant may not work. His comment to me was that Chad and Rachael were not responsible enough for him to be at home for the rest of the regimen. I inquired that if I stayed with him and oversaw the medications and treatments would he let him go home. The doctor agreed that as long as I was with Chad for every moment of his care again during that time he would release him to my care. I went back to Chad's room to let him know that he would be released that day. He thanked me over and over again. Now I would have to start over again instilling hope in Chad.

We finally received word that another donor had been found that was not as compatible as the first but that they thought was close enough to match for the transplant. Time was staring us in the face, straight in the eyes, as Chad seemed to become weaker and sicker as each day passed. He had no other choice but to risk another transplant even if it was not with a perfect donor match.

A date was set and in just weeks they were ready for transplant. The procedure of the transplant from the second donor was accepted well by Chad. There were no complications during the procedure. The following day Chad had to get two units of blood and was started on the Prograf medication once again for possible GVHD. He was now starting to feel good and just a little tired but with a little more positive outlook.

By day three after transplant Chad noticed a blotchy rash on his chest. The doctor's office was contacted and we were instructed to give him an antihistamine and his nausea medication. Chad slept well that night. The following day we were headed to the clinic and Chad became very nauseated. The blotchy rash was now spreading to his arms and back. A biopsy was taken of the rash for GVHD but once again showed no signs of the disease. Over a course of several weeks the rash started to diminish until it was soon gone.

We continued to hold on to hope that remission and recover were just around the next corner or beyond the next mountain.

Chapter 24

Eyes to the Soul

They say you can see a person's soul
You can see who they are as a whole
If you look deeply into their eyes
You can even see past any lies

Your eyes have shown your journey well
As I have watched them I can tell
I have seen anger, almost a hate
When you were given this horrible fate

The haze and dullness of feeling ill
When you knew leukemia could kill
A ray of hope came to your eyes
With each remission relief you did sigh

A bright brilliance along with a smile
When Rachael said she would love you all the while
I have seen sunshine in your eyes
When you heard Kiersten's first little cries

Warmth and softness I have seen
And I have never eyed, just mean
Sadness and pain, I have seen that too
I have even seen them change their hue

But most of the time I see in you eyes
The tender caring love beyond your cries

HOLDING ON FOR DEAR LIFE

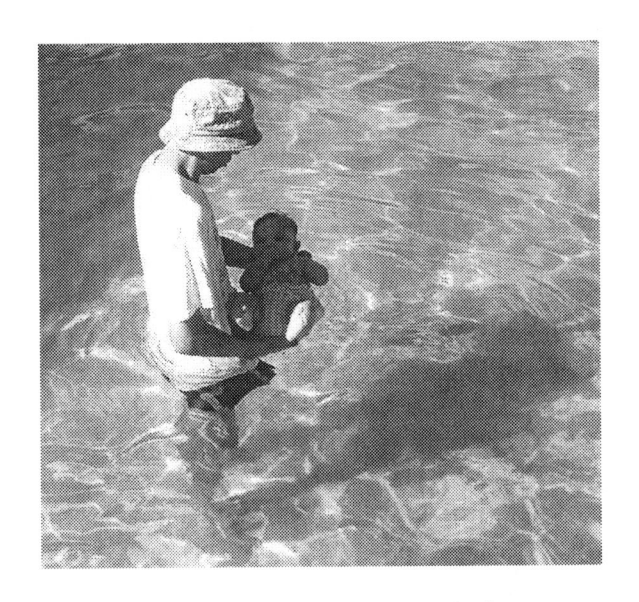

Father/Daughter Pool Time

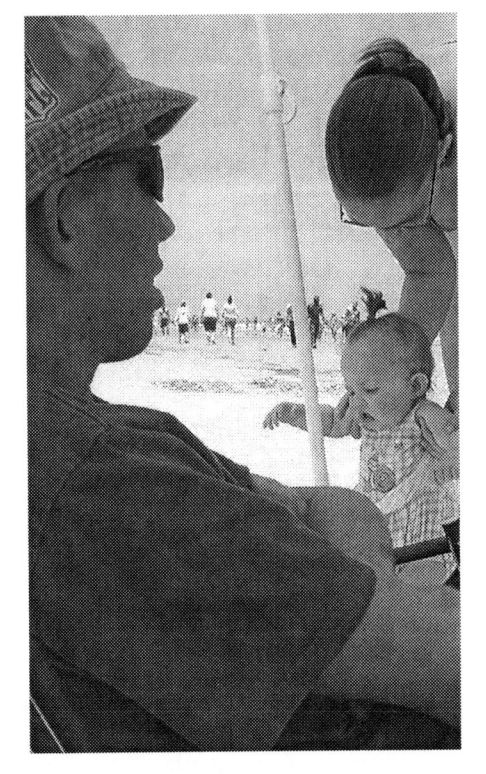

Enjoying Kiersten at the Beach

Chad's father decided to put in for a temporary transfer with his job so that he could be in Atlanta to help Rachael with Chad for a few months. I was glad he had made this decision and welcomed the help for Chad and Rachael. I had lost my job at the chiropractor office because I had been in Atlanta too long so I desperately needed to return home to seek employment.

I returned to Atlanta on February 25th so we could celebrate Chad's twenty-seventh birthday. He was not much in the mood to celebrate as he was running a fever, weak, having some difficulty breathing and was neutropenic from the chemotherapy. A call was made to the doctor; Chad was admitted again into the bone marrow transplant unit at the hospital and placed on oxygen. He needed fluids, blood and platelets that were administered over several days.

A CT scan of his chest revealed that the axillary lump was decreasing in size but a new moderate pericardial effusion was found along with small pleural effusions in both sides of the lung. Pleural effusions are abnormal accumulations of fluid in the pleural space around the lungs that can be malignant. The doctors were questioning fungal pneumonia.

The following day a procedure was done called bronchial washing to Chad's right upper lung lobe and left upper and lower lobes. The findings were verification of fungal organisms, epithelial cells and pneumonia.

This procedure was preceded by a CT of the sinuses and face that revealed generalized cerebral volume loss that was much advanced for his age. Cerebral volume loss is something that is a normal function of the brain as we age and can possibly be associated with epilepsy. An echocardiogram was done that showed insufficiency of the aorta and a small pericardial effusion of the heart. It appeared that Chad's body was aging at a fast steady pace. Chad desperately wanted to be released from the hospital to return home to rest and take his medication. I hated to leave but I had to return home to Savannah.

A few days later Rachael called to inform me of the test results and Chad's condition. She also informed me that the doctors were releasing him to return home from the hospital. Rachael continued to keep me abreast of the latest on how Chad was feeling and what was going on.

Three weeks had passed since my last visit and with each report I was becoming more nervous and concerned. I discussed with Shawn the findings and condition his brother was in. He wanted to see Chad and spend some time with him. Later that evening I called Rachael back to let her know that Shawn, Cathy and I were coming up for a visit.

Chad was always encouraging me to come stay with them and to come up any time and as often and as long a stay as I could. I had talked to him on the phone that afternoon and he seemed to be down in spirit and this concerned me as he was also not feeling his best physically. I knew that a visit from Shawn would be just what he needed. Besides, it had been a three-week stretch since I last visited and seen Kiersten.

Chad was not much in the mood to visit long with anyone when we arrived. He was worn out and tired. His body was weak and again frail. He was beginning to have difficulty walking due to his hip problems. He mostly just wanted to stay in bed and rest. He did express being glad that we had come for a visit. Shawn and Chad did spend as much time visiting as Chad could tolerate and that pleased me.

I had been the main care giver for Chad over the past three and a half years and it seemed to be working well how I was doing it so far. Most of it was giving the encouragement and positive outlook of whatever situation he was facing at the time. Doing this through a deep-seeded mother's love for her child made it easy. As physical times were difficult I would almost cater to him but that is when his body needed the time to rest and heal. That was when he needed the most encouragement. As his health would progress I would start letting him do more for himself as his strength permitted. Often he wanted me to rub his feet or scratch his head. I enjoyed being able to do such a minimal thing as it gave him comfort somehow. You could just see him relax and he needed that desperately.

Whatever way I had been doing to take care of Chad seemed to help him survive his battles to this point in his life. I did not approve of what I felt was a lack of his care by others at times. I wondered sometimes if others just did not realize the true condition Chad was in mentally as well as emotionally and physically. I wondered if sometimes others just did not understand how hard it was for him to do many things for himself for daily living. Rachael and I often questioned and requested a review of Chad's medications and tests. Whatever the cause for his current difficulties, it seemed more imperative than ever to support him emotionally at this time.

Chad was at a point now where he needed daily encouragement. It was difficult and painful for him to even walk due to his hip pain. When he was hungry he would rather go without eating than to have to get up and try and fix something for himself. Emotionally he was becoming tired of the whole battle and needed a loving touch and kind word frequently. Much of his time now seemed to be spent in bed resting. He seemed to be shutting himself in again. Conversation was at a minimum and he was trying to keep to himself a lot of the time. This was breaking my heart.

As my visit came to an end it was difficult for me to see him in the condition he was in and return home. It was a four-and-a-half-hour drive from my front door to their front door; however, it was only forty-five minutes by airplane if I was needed quickly. I reassured Chad that I was not far away if he needed me.

One of the hardest precautions had become very hard to adhere to. As Chad became sicker and in more pain as time passed, he also became more cautious about possible contact with illnesses. If he was even the least bit neutropenic he would be afraid to hold Kiersten or allow anyone to even give him a hug. That was very difficult. When I would arrive for a visit and see how ill and weak he looked I wanted to take him in my arms and just hold him. Because of fear, he would not allow these things to happen. Another reason I hated this thing called leukemia. It was robbing us of precious hugs.

Chad returned to the hospital on March 6th for admission again only eight days later. He was again neutropenic, running a fever intermittently, experiencing an altered mental state, having increasing gastro-intestinal distress, severe weakness, poor appetite and increased sleepiness. He had become forgetful and seemed unable to reason things out and concentrate.

Another CT of the chest confirmed that the pneumonia had become worse in the upper right lobe. It was now scattered and patchy throughout the lungs with ill-defined nodular infiltrates and increased volumes of pleural effusion. An MRM of the brain showed a definite cerebral atrophy that was well advanced for Chad's age. Antibiotics were continued.

More studies were done over the next following weeks that showed that the pericardial effusion was decreasing, the pleural effusion was resolved and there was improvement in the right upper lung lobe. The echocardiogram showed no change to his heart condition.

During Chad's hospital stay the doctor voiced his concern that the bone marrow from the second donor transplant was not growing. This meant that Chad's body was setting with very little cells and what was there were very likely going to be the leukemia cells. There were no signs of GVHD that could be found. His body was not fighting any foreign cells.

An attempt was made to contact the second donor to do a third transplant. It was never made clear to us as to if the donor refused to donate again or if it was that the donor could not be contacted. Either way it was evident that Chad was in deep dark trouble.

For a back-up plan the doctors still had another bag of the very first donor's stem cells that had been stored. It was with hopes of bringing the GVHD into effect and the bone marrow to grow. His medications were also evaluated and readjusted which seemed to help with the confusion and mental difficulties. Chad was released to return home once again.

I was not aware of the severity of Chad's condition or all that had been going on during this period of time. I was concerned that Chad felt that I had deserted him even though I did call him often. It was difficult talking to him as he was so ill, his mind confused and he just wanted to sleep most of the time. He was not able to tell me what all was going on with him or what the doctors were saying. At times when I spoke with him it was difficult for him to carry on any normal conversation and his voice was soft and weak making it difficult to understand him.

I had been talking on the phone frequently with Jeremy and Joshua to keep them up on what I knew of Chad's condition. They had become very concerned of his becoming so ill again. They decided it was time for them to take a road trip to Atlanta from the Midwest. Jeremy, Joshua and his wife, Melissa, made the trip down to see Chad.

It was difficult for them to see Chad in the condition that he was in. The last time they had seen and been around Chad was when he was still his fun-loving, outgoing self at his and Rachael's wedding. Now he was mentally and physically worn down. He had lost a lot of weight and his mind was still not functioning as it totally should.

Chad was thrilled to have them there to spend time with but it was difficult for him to really visit. He was going to the clinic for daily visits and that also interfered with their time together. When he would return from his clinic visits he was worn out and wanted to take a nap. However, for Chad's mind, it was emotionally uplifting for him to have them care enough to make that journey to see him.

After visiting Chad for two days they ventured on to Savannah to see Shawn, Cathy and myself. They learned firsthand of why Chad had an inner desire to relocate. Savannah's charm and style took our visitors by surprise and won their hearts. I was glad they had made the trip on down to see us. After seeing the condition Chad was in it was important for them to be able to talk about it and voice their concern. An evening on River Street and a little beach combing and it was time for them to depart. A day later they were headed back to Atlanta to see Chad once more before their trip back to Kansas. When I spoke with Chad I learned that it had done his self-esteem good to have them visit. His voice sounded a little more perky now.

During the time away from Atlanta I searched for other options of alternative treatments that were available for the possibilities for Chad's recovery in his battle for life. I was not alone in my search. Several of my friends and family members sent suggestions to me of treatments they had heard about.

My friend Elaine in Oklahoma was constantly searching for options and spent much time researching what she could. She had known Chad since his birth and was more like family to us than a friend. She was more like a sister to me and the boys knew her as Aunt Elaine. Elaine had been a constant source of support for me from the beginning of Chad's battle. During times that I did not have the time to research something, she was there doing it for me.

Most of the places I contacted about treatments they offered would not be accepted by Chad's insurance and were extremely costly. We were limited to what types of treatment we could try. Yes, life is priceless but most of these places of treatment wanted cash up front since it was not covered by insurance. That is the price of some research.

We would all continue to do all we could that was feasible to get Chad well and try and keep him out of the hospital as much as possible. The doctor became open to the possibility of sending Chad to other bigger research center hospitals for other options. He doubted they would do anything different than what he was doing. He himself had been in contact with several other doctors to get their opinions and help. None of us were ready to give up helping Chad with his battle because we all wanted to keep Chad in our lives.

Chapter 25
April 2004

Love

Love is a thing
That can make a heart sing
It can make you cry awhile
But it can make you smile

Love is a really beautiful thing
Joy to you it can bring
It makes you do things you have never done before
It can give you strength and make your heart soar

Love is for sharing
Just to let you know someone is caring
It comes with ups and downs
And also laughs and frowns

Love is a gift of giving
It makes it all worth living
A brighter future you will see
If you can say, not I, but we

Love can give such happy things
A gift from God to you it brings
Each day it grows a little stronger
As you hold on a little longer

DEBBI HUFF

Love will never end they say
It will always pass your way
If you can open up your heart
It can become a working gift of art

My love for you grows day to day
But this scares me, in a way
I love you so very much
I never want to miss your touch

I pray to God in Heaven above
That I shall never lose your love

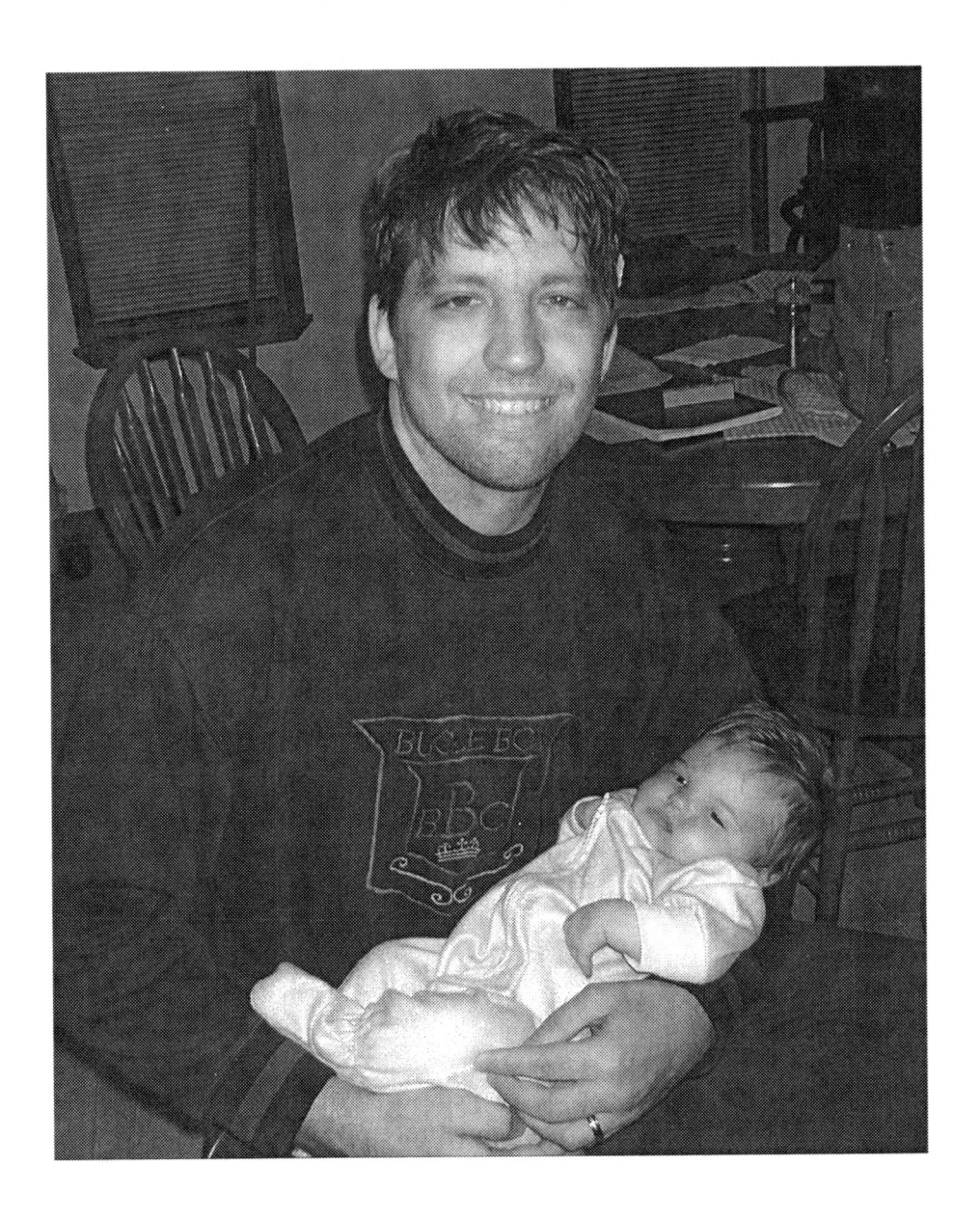

Chad and Kiersten

With Chad back home he was once again with the routine visits to the clinic. A follow-up bone marrow biopsy was done on April thirtieth. The result showed an increased amount of iron but was clean of any cancer. Medication was given to decrease his high iron level.

For the next two months several CT scans and x-rays of Chad's chest were done periodically. Sometime they showed improvement and sometimes they showed continuous problems.

In June another blood culture was done with results showing there were no viruses found. Chad was finally overcoming this obstacle. He was once again pushing back the enemy lines.

A workup was done during the months of June and July. Another bone marrow biopsy showed to be clean. A CT of the chest showed improvement was continuing in the lungs, a CT of the abdomen and pelvis showed no problems, a CT of the testicle showed normal with no masses, a bronchi alveolar lavage showed no cancer or viral problems in the lungs, a chest x-ray showed the heart to be of borderline in size with no changes, a whole body bone scan showed no problems, and a testing of the cerebrospinal fluid showed no cancer growth. An x-ray of the hips still showed bilateral femoral head avascular necroses with stable mild subchondral collapse of the right femoral head.

It looked as though Chad could once again start getting his life back to a more normal state except for the hip pain that he experienced due to the degenerative disease. All tests showed improvement but Chad still remained tired and weak.

The triple IV catheter was removed from the left side of Chad's chest giving him more of a sense of freedom from all this madness. All was going well and we all felt that Chad was no longer in danger as he slowly progressed.

Chad was now becoming more active and feeling some better. He was becoming more involved with events of the outside world. He talked often of how he and Rachael had gone to see Atlanta's baseball team play and how he wanted to go see another one and take me to a game. Just as I had always been excited to show him new experiences he was now becoming excited to show me new experiences.

Chad was always active in sports. He had played on baseball teams every summer of his younger years. Starting with t-ball and working up to regular baseball. The last year he played he was catcher. He loved being on his soccer team, participating in bicycle races, shooting bow and arrows, wrestling, golfing, and had advanced well towards a black belt in taekwondo. As the years passed on to high school days he still remained interested in sports but declined playing them so much.

Mid-June I was on my way home from work and was involved in a seven car pile up. My SUV was totaled as I was sandwiched between vehicles. I was off from work for six weeks and unable to drive. Chad and Rachael came to stay with us for a few days to help me as I was unable to do many of life's functions due to my injuries. Chad was always a family-oriented person and there to help in any way he could when needed. He put his own problems and difficulties aside to come be of help in any way he could. Seldom did he let his own illness keep him from showing his loving kindness.

My friend Lisa, from Missouri, came out with Great Uncle Archie to spend the Fourth of July weekend with us. Lisa returned after the weekend and my great uncle stayed on with me for six weeks. As I gradually recovered from my injuries he kept me company. Once I was recovered we made a trip to Atlanta so that he could see Chad and visit with him for a few days.

In August Chad and Rachael and Kiersten came down for a visit. During this visit we went to the beach to see the sand sculptures that were made for a sand sculpture contest. It was Kiersten's first time to be at the beach and get her feet in the sand and the ocean. Chad was pleased to see that she was going to love the beach and water as much as he did.

As the months passed, the doctors continued with their poking and prodding to monitor Chad's condition. Results continued to show stability and improvement. We all seemed to be getting back into the normal routine of life once again. I went to Atlanta occasionally for visits and Chad and Rachael came to Savannah when they could.

By October twenty-eighth the CT of the chest showed the lungs well expanded and no new findings. Blood cultures continued to come back with no new growth.

Chad started talking about wanting to move to the Savannah area. I contacted the cancer clinic in Savannah and Chad's doctor in Atlanta. Chad's doctor knew the doctors in Savannah and gave his approval for Chad to make the move. The clinic in Savannah said they had no problem with keeping Chad's doctor in Atlanta abreast of anything that would be going on with Chad and working with him on his treatments. Rachael was not ready to make a move yet at that time due to her job so the move was placed on hold for the future.

In November Chad noticed a wound starting to become evident on his left great toe. It seemed to be getting worse as the days passed. Upon having a culture done the doctors found staphylococcus aureus infection. Antibiotics were ordered and administered with success.

At the same time there was concern of redness about Chad's IV port. Because of possible infection at the port site it was removed from the side of Chad's chest and a temporary catheter was inserted into his left arm. This would still give access for treatments without him continually being stuck with a needle with each clinic visit and would be easily removed when treatments were completed.

Chad was looking forward to celebrating Kiersten's first birthday. It was a small celebration with ten of us at their home and some being young, under the age of ten. Chad remained seated on the couch to keep his distance from the children until it was time for the cake and ice cream. There was some concern about him being around small children since he still had not been revaccinated for childhood illnesses. It was wonderful seeing the pride and joy in his face as his little girl indulged in cake and ice cream on her own. She ended up with more of it on her than in her as we all laughed.

We looked back at Kiersten's first year. She had learned to roll over, sit up, crawl, walk, laugh, play and started to talk. Her first words were "da-da." There were so many new things she had learned to do.

As the year was nearing to a close we looked forward to a more positive new year ahead. CT scans and x-rays still held steady with improvement with no signs of cancer or viral infections.

During one of Chad's visits to the clinic we were told by the doctor that Chad was well in remission from the leukemia and it was only a matter of several weeks now before they did hip replacement surgery. He then stated that after Chad recovered from his hip surgery he would be ready to go back to work and start living a normal life again. We were thrilled of the news. After all this long battle he was finally going to come out the winner.

Christmas would be a time of joy in our family. This Christmas we would get to have our little family all together to celebrate. It would be Kiersten's first Christmas to be old enough to start enjoying her gifts. It was one of those times that everything seemed to be coming to an end with Chad's battle and would be with a good outcome. There would be a new beginning and new life ahead for him.

Then once again my phone rang.

Chapter 26
December 2004

God's Love Can Show

Love, there will be a new day
It may be near or far away
If it be in Heaven
Or if it be on earth
Only God does know

Heart, you will feel no more sadness
An end will come to all this madness
Be it in silence
Or be it in loudness
Only God does know

Mind, why be so jumbled up inside
Are you not looking to confide
Is it only a mind game
Am I still not me, one and the same
Only God does know

Body, you show beyond time in years
Can you just walk me through this land of tears
Will you drop and fall
Or around my heart will you build a wall
Only God does know

Tears, must you roll and fall
Are you really so sad to call
Must you fill these eyes
I do not want to have any more cries
Only God does know

Eyes, will you sparkle any day now
Did you forget just how
Will you close away
Or will you try to shine today
Only God does know

Mouth, must you always turn down
It is so tiring to frown
Will you go on forever
Or will I smile again never
Only God does know

God, please hear me now
Answer my prayers somehow
Let my heart sing
Let my mind be at ease
Let my body stand strong
Let my tears fall only in gladness
Let my eyes see only beauty
Let my mouth smile with joy
Let my love grow on and on
So I may show the love You give
And how through You I did live

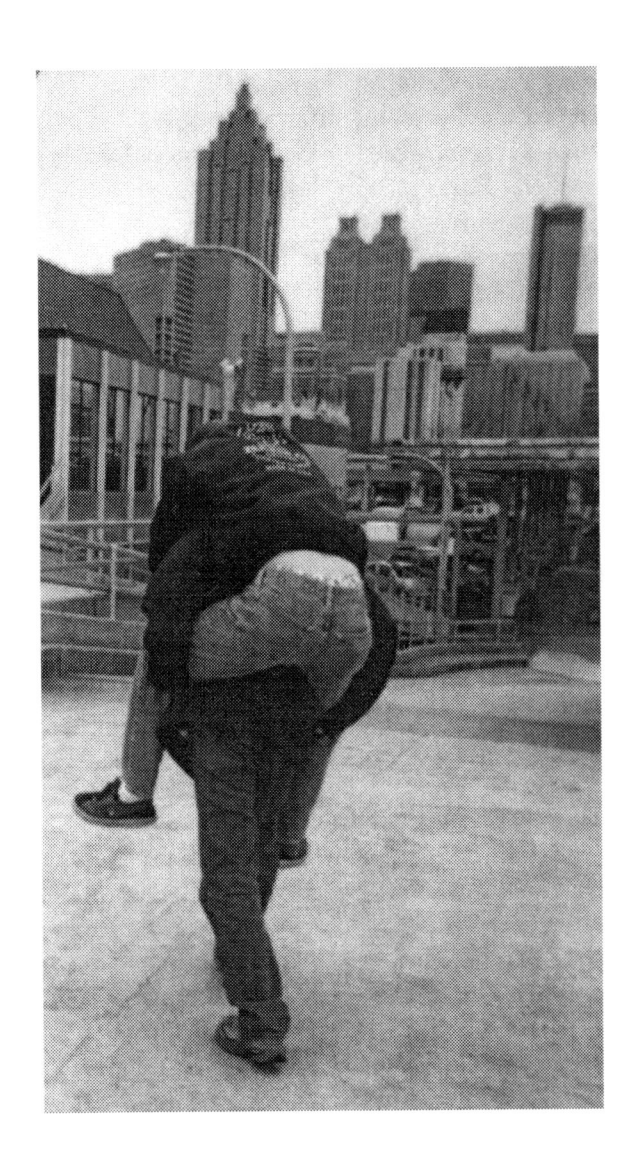

A Brother's Helping Hand in Time of Need
Shawn and Chad in Atlanta

Mid-December I received a call from Rachael that once again caught me off guard. Chad had started having difficulty breathing and was taken to the hospital. After several studies the doctors discovered fluid around his lungs and heart.

Immediate surgery was done to place two chest tubes with a drain to drain off the fluid. One tube was to drain the fluid from around his lungs and the other to drain fluid from around his heart. This was very painful for Chad to endure even with the medications.

The findings of fungal pneumonia had reared its ugly head once again and this time wasted no time in getting the upper hand.

Antibiotics and intravenous fluids were administered. He was placed on oxygen to make it easier for him to breathe. He was kept as comfortable as they possibly could keep him with medication. He was placed on a diuretic medication to help his body get rid of any extra fluid that was building up. When the tubes were finally removed he started showing signs of improvement. I returned home to finish arrangements for Christmas.

Chad was able to be out of the hospital in time for Christmas. However, plans for the location of our celebration were now changed to Atlanta. He would be unable to make the trip to Savannah. The location made us no difference as long as we were together as a family to celebrate.

Upon completing my work shift on Christmas day, I drove to Atlanta with gifts, warmth in my heart and a smile on my face. Shawn and Cathy would be following and arriving later that night after they got off work.

Chad was once again on daily visits to the clinic so the morning started off with an all-too-familiar routine. Once again it seemed he had regressed but hope was not lost. This was just a small hurdle for him to overcome. He had been doing well and his health seemed to be improving enough to help fight off any infections.

After his clinic visit, the day after Christmas, we returned to the house to celebrate and open gifts. Chad was not in his upbeat mood that day. He was hurting and exhausted. He did the best he could to be positive but spent much of the day resting and visiting with Shawn. The two did spend a short time outside running their battery powered race cars that they both enjoyed. They talked of how they were going to race them together at the different tracks and how they could make them faster and of course which one of them had the faster car to beat the other.

It was becoming very difficult for Chad to walk with the progression of the degenerative hip disease so Great Uncle Archie and I purchased a hand-carved cane for him to use. It worked well for getting about for short distances but Chad now needed a wheelchair for any distances farther than a walk to the bedroom from the living room or to the car. Stairs became almost unbearable with pain for him to manage. My heart ached for him with each painful step he felt. He had to maneuver stairs to get out of the house or to even go to the car in the garage in the house they were living in.

Rachael voiced concern of managing their funds to me. We had both tapped what was left of our funds and living dollar to dollar. Chad was once again on visits to the clinic three times a week. Rachael was trying to juggle working and taking care of Kiersten and Chad. It was all becoming too overwhelming for her.

A week after Christmas Rachael called me and asked if I could move back in with them and help with Chad and Kiersten. He would need someone with him continually for several weeks after he had his hip surgery. I did not have to be asked twice. I immediately started making plans of how I would make the move.

I promptly started making plans. By this time I was working full time for an airline. I went in and spoke with my manager at work and after explaining the situation she said she would check with our center in Atlanta to see if they would agree to a transfer. I then started checking on finding a storage unit facility. I did not think twice about putting my things in storage once again. At no time over the past few years had I carried any regrets or resentments for the material things that I released. There were also no regrets over the financial problems I had and was now facing or the major changes that were happening frequently in my personal life. With each time I moved my belongings I was able to part with some things which eventually left me with little to move. The clutter had been cleared out. I learned the difference of knowing what you need and knowing what you want and the importance of both. I learned that material things are just that. One does not have to have the biggest or best to be happy. The important thing in life is life itself with trust and faith in the Lord.

The reservation center in Atlanta was in agreement with the transfer so I began packing my belongings. They also agreed to me working the evening shift so I could be with Chad and Kiersten to care for them through the day while Rachael was at work. After making final arrangements and placing the last item in storage, Whiskers and I were on our way to make our new home with Chad, Rachael and Kiersten. As with the other house they had previously lived in, they made sure this one had a mom's room too. This room was now referred to as grandma's room, however. I would begin my first day at the Atlanta center on Monday, January 10th. Shawn and Cathy had gotten them a place of their own to live so all seemed to be working out well for housing arrangements on such short notice.

By mid February, Rachael got a shower chair for Chad to use. Taking a shower or bath also was now becoming difficult with stepping in and out of the shower and the risk of slipping. It was difficult for Chad to stand for long periods of time and his patience was becoming short towards himself for his shortcomings.

One evening Chad asked me instead of Rachael for the first time to help assist him for a shower. Rachael had always been the one to assist him before but she was gone. As I helped him remove his sweat suit my heart sank and I gulped back the tears. I knew all Chad's body had gone through since his battle began but it stared me in the face now. He had scars on his body from where the breast biopsies had been done, on both sides of his upper chest where the IV catheters and port had been, the scar from when they had inserted the filter to keep blood clots from going to his upper body, and two long scars from where the chest tubes had been inserted. There were scars on his hips from all the bone marrow biopsies that had been done and the spinal punctures he had been through. There were leftover telltale discolored areas from where the dark dime-sized cancer had reared its head. I knew he had scars also from the removal of the testicle and from a surgery to remove his appendix when he was a child.

His body that was usually covered by a sweat suit or hospital gown had kept covered a body that was frail in appearance with mostly just skin over bone with little fat on it now. By now he had lost most of his upbeat humor and smile. He was becoming tired of the battle and his spirits were low.

The doctor had informed us that he would need to delay Chad's scheduling for his hip replacement surgery out by about six more months. He had to first recover from the fungal pneumonia and chest tube surgery. The delay only frustrated Chad more.

Lisa once again made plans to come out to visit from Missouri. She would be arriving a week after my move to Atlanta to help with what she could. It was a welcome visit, as always.

Since Lisa was coming to visit we had moved an old living room rocker chair from "Grandma's" bedroom to the living room before her arrival so there would be plenty of seating. The chair was a little wobbly but if you sat carefully it would not tip.

Rachael was on the couch and I was seated on the loveseat watching television when Chad came from their bedroom to join us in the living room. He decided to sit in the chair. We had encouraged him to sit on the couch or love seat but he wanted to sit in the chair. He had seated himself comfortably when Whiskers saw it inviting to jump onto the back of it to sit. This was a common sitting place for Whiskers at home on my recliner. As soon as Whiskers jumped onto the back of the chair it tipped backwards. With hearing a short yell, Rachael and I turned to see the chair on the floor and Chad's feet sticking straight up in the air. We were all laughing so hard that we had difficulty getting the chair upright for Chad to get up. Needless to say he sat on the couch after that encounter.

The following Sunday after work I stopped by the airport to pick up Lisa at the airport. It was good to see her and I knew with her upbeat cheerfulness she would be good for Chad to be around for awhile. Lisa had become part of my rock of support. Often she had been out to visit, either by airplane or driving. It was always good for me to have her there.

On Tuesday January 18th Lisa went with Chad and me to the clinic for his bone marrow biopsy, lab work and CT scan of his chest and sinuses that showed improvement. Between the two of them they kept me laughing and my bubbly personality started showing itself again after being hidden for so long. I had not realized how serious and introverted I had started becoming. Lisa had brought a few days of much-needed sunshine and laughter with her visit into our lives.

But as we had learned from the past, anything can change at a moment's notice.

Chapter 27

No Tomorrow Guaranteed

Count your blessing each and every day
You never know when tomorrow will go away
Laugh each day instead of pout
Say I love you without a doubt

For in case tomorrow does not come
Regrets, you may have some
Say you are sorry where you must
Before ashes to ashes and dust to dust

Tomorrow is no guarantee
And in the end we all pay a fee
Do not be left standing outside Heaven's shore
Or at the entrance to the fiery door

On Wednesday Chad slept most of the day. I went in occasionally to check on him. With some concern in my heart, I went in and spoke with him about taking Lisa to the airport for her departure and going on to work that afternoon. He said he was fine and to go on. I knew Rachael would be home within the following hour. I took Lisa back to the airport on my way to work for her return back to Missouri.

That evening I received a disturbing phone call at work from Rachael. When she had returned home Chad was still sleeping. She checked in on him occasionally and a little later she went it to wake him for their evening meal. She could barely get him to respond to her. Chad had become lethargic, his muscles seemed to be twitching and he was unable to control his movements enough to even sit on the side of the bed.

She told me that she had called the doctor and was instructed to take him to the emergency room. Chad was unable to cooperate mentally or physically to get himself out of the bed. Rachael was trying to handle him and Kiersten to get them all three to the car. I suggested she call the ambulance immediately and then call me back.

The next call I received was to let me know that the ambulance was on its way and that she would meet me at the emergency entrance of the hospital. She told me that Chad was somewhat combative with the ambulance attendants but due to lack of control and strength they had no difficulty with transporting him.

I wasted no time in explaining the situation to my supervisor and departed for the hospital immediately. Upon my transfer from Savannah, my previous supervisor had made the Atlanta office aware of the situation that was the reason for the transfer. All the staff in the Atlanta office were understanding and cooperative.

The next call I received from Rachael was alarming. She called me to let me know that she thought the ambulance was headed to the wrong hospital. There were two hospitals in North Atlanta with the same name. She was in pursuit behind them but was having difficulty keeping up with them. Then she lost staying behind them when they went through the red light with siren blasting.

I was already in the hospital parking lot so I went into the emergency room to inquire of the ambulance arrival. I approached the receptionist desk with fear and anxiety rushing through me. They did have word that there was an ambulance coming in but no specifics on with whom or where it was coming from. They were unable to tell me if it was the ambulance that was transporting Chad.

I returned a call to Rachael to let her know that they had no idea. It seemed as though I waited for hours and my heart raced with every ambulance that pulled up in front of the emergency room only to find out it was not the one Chad was in. I feared that if they took him to the wrong hospital he would not get the appropriate care because they did not have a cancer center. I feared that they would not make it to the hospital in time and Chad might lose his life in an ambulance.

Finally I received a welcome phone call. Rachael called that the ambulance was on its way to the correct hospital but that it had taken the longer route instead of the shorter one and should be there shortly.

Upon their arrival I could not see Chad as they took him in through a back entrance. I met with Rachael in the hospital parking lot and took over tending to Kiersten so that she could go back and be with Chad in the examination room. We both wanted desperately to find out what condition he was in and what was going on in his tired, weak body.

In the emergency room they immediately did an overall assessment of Chad and ordered a CAT scan of the brain, a chest x-ray and lab work. They were unable to determine what the cause was. He was then admitted to the bone marrow transplant unit in the hospital.

Once in the unit his doctor arrived and ordered blood cultures, a urinary catheter, and an intravenous infusion with three different antibiotics. Chad was now semi-conscious with his eyes twitching and moving his mouth as if talking but with no or little sound coming out. If anyone touched his skin he would let out a cry as if it caused him severe pain.

Finally around five in the morning he seemed to be resting with no twitching but was yawning quite frequently. When I would try and speak with him he still gave no response to where he was or who I was. He would look at me with a blank stare that made me wonder if he even recognized me at all. He had now also started running a fever.

The CAT scan results came back normal and the blood levels were all in normal range so the doctor decided to do an MRI of Chad's brain and a lumbar puncture with insertion of chemotherapy.

When Chad was returned to his room after the lumbar puncture the twitching had returned along with jerking motions. Now he seemed to be yawning almost constantly. The doctor arrived a little later to say that the lumbar puncture findings were also normal. Everyone was puzzled as to what was going on. It was a long night with little sleep as I stayed at Chad's beside so Rachael could take Kiersten home to put her to bed and try to get some rest herself.

The following morning another doctor was on call that examined Chad and said he thought it to be from all the drugs Chad was on. This was the same doctor that had belittled Chad about missing his dose of chemotherapy. He ordered a shot to be given that would clean any drugs out of Chad's system. The doctor, nurse and I observed as we saw no change in Chad's condition from the injection. This showed that what was going on in Chad's body had nothing to do with the drugs they had prescribed. The doctor then ordered a feeding tube be placed for nutrition. The doctors were at awe of what was causing these reactions and symptoms in Chad.

Rachael arrived at the hospital the following morning to see Chad as soon as she had gotten herself and Kiersten fed and dressed for the day. When Chad heard her voice he tried to talk to her. Still little or no sound came from his mouth and what did was weak. She reached her hand out to his and he clutched her thumb and did not want to let go. He needed her there for comfort. He seemed to rest much better after her arrival. Often Chad spoke to me of how much he loved Rachael and that he did not know what he would do without her by his side.

Later that day Chad started chilling and became restless after the feeding tube was placed and was voicing curse words. Once again the all-too-familiar fear of my son possibly dying passed through my body. I thought of all he had been through and how he had already been through so much both mentally and physically. I thought about how much he loved us to continue this battle and search for strength when he was so weak.

I sat back in the chair at his bedside and thought of how this was not how this story I was writing was supposed to end. I wanted it to end with him being healthy again, in remission, going to college, pursuing a career, meeting his first transplant donor as a survivor and growing old to watch Kiersten mature into a beautiful young lady. I began to pray and search for my strength in my faith. Chad had shown his strength and courage before when his doctors had given up on his survival. I expected no less from him again this time. Once again I prayed for Michael to come with his army of angels to help Chad with this new battle.

Shortly after four in the afternoon Chad raised his arms into the air, started yelling, and threw his head back as his eyes rolled back in his head and then stared without blinking. I immediately yelled for a nurse. Chad's nurse came in promptly and had me help to turn Chad onto his side. He said it appeared that Chad was having a seizure. The doctor arrived quickly and ordered medication that would help Chad to relax. A neurologist was called in and he placed Chad on medication for seizures and ordered a STAT MRI. An oxygen cannula was placed into Chad's nostrils. After a short time he seemed to be resting in a more relaxed and peaceful state.

With fear in my voice and a shaking hand I picked up the phone and called Rachael, my mother and father and Shawn to let them know of this turn of events. I attempted to get a flight for Shawn and Cathy to arrive as soon as possible but was unable to due to times of flights out of Savannah. Rachael informed me that she would be on her way up to the hospital and Shawn and Cathy would be arriving early the following morning. My parents would be praying for Chad and inform other family members of the events.

Rachael found a sitter for Kiersten and arrived shortly after my call to her. Upon her arrival the medical staff was trying to get an EEG of Chad's brainwaves but were unable to obtain an accurate reading. Chad's temperature had risen and he was sweating too much for the wire leads to stay on. Chad was then taken down to get the MRI done that had been ordered. Rachael and I both accompanied him for this procedure.

Upon returning to Chad's hospital room we were informed that they found out that the chest x-ray showed that the feeding tube had not been placed properly. It was then reinserted with another x-ray to follow. Chad remained restless and gagging on phlegm. He had to be suctioned frequently and I was told I could suction him if I saw him choking. I had to place a chair to sit in by the head of his bed as the suctioning was almost constant. After a short time of this the feeding tube was removed. Upon removal, the gagging and suctioning stopped. Chad seemed to calm down and rest better now.

The infectious disease doctor had been contacted to come see Chad. He arrived that evening and upon his examination he determined a diagnosis of possible meningitis. The doctors were all still just speculating. Chad was placed on antibiotics.

Shawn and Cathy drove to Atlanta and arrived very early the following morning. It was difficult for Shawn to see Chad in such a condition. I can still visualize Chad lying in the hospital bed with Shawn adorned in a yellow disposable gown and blue shoe covers (a must to enter the BMT Unit). He was standing at the foot of the hospital bed with tears rolling down his cheeks. Shawn's whole body was trembling. This whole ordeal had been so hard for him to handle. I thanked God that he had Cathy by his side to comfort him at the times I could not be there with him.

Shawn questioned me as to how I could handle all this. I had never thought about that until then. How was I able to handle all this? At times I did not know. Yes, it was very, very difficult for me to see him go through these hard times. My times of tears behind closed doors were frequent. But when with him I would fight the tears back because my love for him was so great that I was not about to depart his side through the hard times when he needed me most. Chad was handling much worse than I ever was both physically and mentally. What I was feeling in this storm of his life was just a minute speck in the massive sea of turmoil to what he was feeling, thinking and going through. He needed me and so I was there. Through my faith I was finding the strength and whatever else it was I was needing to help get Chad through this without totally losing it myself.

Our prayers were answered a week later when Chad recovered and was able to return home. Once again when the doctors had all but given up on him surviving, he responded with the miracle of life. He progressed slowly each day and we took all the positive advances he could get. Once again Chad had removed a mountain from his road to recovery. It still left puzzlement as to what had happened to Chad and no definite diagnosis was ever determined.

Upon our returning back to the house we got a good night's sleep. That following morning I thought about what Shawn had asked me. I took a long look at myself in the mirror. I felt and thought that I looked like I had aged twenty years in a short time. I looked at the new wrinkles that had found their way onto my thinning face and the thinning of my hair. Lord, I thought in silent prayer, I know you only put before us what we can handle with Your help but please let Chad stay well now. He has had enough hard times and hurts for this lifetime and the next. I once again drew my strength from faith and prepared to start the day.

As I entered the living room and saw Chad it was as though my eyes were opened to reality. There sat Chad seated on the couch in pain not only physically but also in his heart. I realized how frail and fragile he had become over this last episode of sickness. He had lost an abundance of weight and his eyes looked tired and sunken. There was not even a glimpse of a sparkle in them. I felt guilty that I had just been feeling sorry for myself after looking in the mirror. God forgive me for my self concern, I thought to myself as I prayed it to God. My thoughts then returned to Chad. We would have to get him eating more again to gain strength and weight. Much support and comfort care was needed again now with encouragement.

Rachael had received information in the mail about a national company holding a baby beauty pageant and we decided we would give it a try. Perhaps it would help raise the spirits of a beaten-down daddy. No matter where we were with Kiersten there was always someone that commented about how beautiful she was. She looked just like Chad at that same age. I had heard on the radio about a baby contest at a well-known local department store also. We decided to enter Kiersten in it as a practice run. Chad wanted to go even though it would be a long day and would tire him out badly.

That morning we loaded Chad and his wheelchair, Kiersten and her stroller and Rachael and I into the minivan. There was a long line of parents with children for the contest so I was glad that we had brought the wheelchair for Chad. We signed Kiersten up even though she did not understand what was going on. Even if Kiersten did not win, it was a fun thing and you could see the pride on Chad's face. That is what made it all worth the time and effort.

With Chad back on a slow but steady road to recovery we all once again had a positive outlook. He was beginning to gain his weight back, although very slowly. He was started on physical therapy to help him build back his strength. His doctor informed us that due to his last illness he would be setting the date for the hip replacement surgery back again by six months. Again this was upsetting and disappointing to Chad, but understandable. Chad had just come through a very life-threatening encounter once again and it would take a little while to recover completely from it all.

Chapter 28
February 2005

A Battle Won

I was not ready for the fight
My future was just looking bright
Leukemia is what the doctor said
With heavy heart I hung my head

My body became an enemy to me
Someone else I wanted to be
The tests and surgeries day after day
At times made me want to run away

But in the end the battle was won
Past dark clouds I found the sun
Cancer would not get the better of me
The battle won, I was now free

Everything was finally continuing on its course for Chad to start his new life after his hip surgery would be completed. We were all settling in on new beginnings once again. We all got a "do over." Chad was still slow to gain weight as we continued to feed him as much as he would tolerate. I would stay on with Chad and Rachael for awhile longer to make sure things were on a good uphill climb.

Once again there were glimpses in our lives for laughter and special moments. One afternoon, while Rachael was at work, Chad, Kiersten and I were in the living room. Chad was seated on the couch and I on the love seat. Kiersten was now fifteen months old, walking, trying to talk and keeping us well entertained with her little antics. I could see a part of Chad in her as her personality began to develop. She had become fascinated with brightly colored beaded necklaces. She would put as many on as she could find around her neck and then prance around the living room.

That very afternoon she did just that again. At one point she had bent over to pick something up off the floor and one of the necklaces went behind her foot as she stepped forward. As she tried to stand up straight the necklace would catch behind her knee making it impossible for her to stand up straight. She was becoming quite frustrated. Her frustration increased as Chad and I laughed until we had tears running down our faces. Eventually I got over to her to help her out of her predicament. She seemed to have Chad's built in knack for making people laugh and perhaps some of his temperament at times. Chad enjoyed watching her grow as she kept him entertained at the same time. She was his sunshine and reason for arising each morning and continuing his battle.

The week of Chad's twenty-eighth birthday was a busy one for him. He was scheduled to see a neurologist, had a dentist appointment, an eye appointment and also a visit to the clinic.

For his birthday we went shopping and I let Chad get new clothes to help prepare for his new beginnings in life after he would have his hip replacement. He was excited and enjoyed getting to select new street clothes. He had been living pretty much in sweats and tee shirts ever since his first bone marrow transplant for comfort and warmth. Due to the pain and difficulty of trying to move from his degenerative hip disease, Rachael had to help him try on his clothes. Even something that simple had become difficult. That evening was a celebration with an ice cream cake. That was Chad's preference to regular cake and ice cream over the past few years.

Once again everything seemed to finally be coming to a closure on this four-year nightmare. It finally looked as if the battle was coming to an end and Chad was going to come out victorious. Once again I thanked God for letting him be here for another birthday, age twenty-eight. One more year he had survived the horrible wounds of his battle.

Chad's doctor had set up an appointment with another neurologist upon request of Rachael and me. The seizure medication seemed to be causing more problems for Chad in regards to shakiness and sleepiness. On the day of the appointment Rachael had to work. I took the minivan and loaded Kiersten with her stroller and Chad with his wheelchair. We were off for an adventure.

We arrived at the parking garage beside the hospital and entered in. The handicap parking spot I finally found in the clinic parking garage was some distance from the front door of the building. I first helped Chad into his wheelchair and locked it beside the van. Next I proceeded to get Kiersten and place her securely in her stroller. We were quite the procession. Chad pushed the stroller and I pushed the wheelchair. That is until we came to a downhill incline in the parking garage to get to the front door of the clinic. I had one hand on the wheelchair on my left side and one hand on the stroller on my right side. I thought, *Okay, God, I can do this.* It was a challenge to keep up with the two wheeled vehicles and keep them going straight at the same time. By the time we reached the walkway to the front entrance of the building Chad and I were bursting with laughter. Kiersten was all smiles as she thought it was fun. Once in the building waiting for the elevator I thought about how we would be going uphill to return to the van. *Lord, give me the strength,* I said silently in my head.

With Chad's appointment came an order for an EEG so that the doctor could determine if Chad truly needed to be on seizure medication. The doctor stated that it was totally up to us if he continued on the medication until the test results came back, but that he recommended he did. We decided to go with this new doctor's decision. The doctor changed the dosage to a lesser amount until the results of the EEG would be obtained.

Now for the trip back to the van. It was a slow steady process. Chad pushed Kiersten, I pushed the wheelchair and we went crosswise up the incline to the minivan. Chad praised me graciously and teased me with joy that this "old woman" was able to do such a feat.

On occasion Chad and Shawn would team up to remind me, teasingly, that I was getting older. Yet they would often tell me that I did not look old like most other women of the same age. They both were outspoken if they would see me wearing anything that would give an "old woman" appearance to my physique. The two of them, along with Jeremy and Joshua, had plans for Tina and me when we became old. They were going to put us in a double room together in a nursing home so we could drive the nursing staff crazy. They were going to fix us up with hot rod motorized wheelchairs so we could have races down the hall.

We arrived at the minivan without a scratch or mishap. The teasing continued with one more comment. I laughed and asked him if he wanted to stop for something to eat on the way home. He then joked about our little outing and how I had worked up an appetite.

Once everyone was loaded, including their wheels of transportation, a thought came to my mind. Why had I not just gotten the minivan and driven down by the front door to pick them up? Needless to say I did not mention this to Chad as he would have really had fun teasing me about that. In reality he was probably thinking the same thing but was kind enough not to say it. A stop at a drive-thru food place and we returned to the house. After eating it was nap time for us all.

To Chad's delight I informed him that I had received a call from my parents while he was sleeping. I told him that they were going to be coming out for a visit to see him. They would be arriving on Thursday. His eyes lit up with happiness. He treasured getting to see family and friends since he could not travel to see them most of the time. The idea of his grandparents traveling halfway across the country to see him lightened his burdens that were lying on his heart. It was hard on Chad not to get to see family as he loved to travel and have new adventures. Now, as often over the past four years, he was unable to travel. The few times he did travel since diagnosis were very hard on him physically.

The Thursday came for my parents' arrival and I went to the airport to pick them up. It was wonderful to get hugs from my mother and father and I was so very glad that they had made the trip to come see Chad. They too were anxious to see him. We had a three-day trip planned to Savannah, at Chad's request, so that they could see Shawn and Cathy and the sights of Savannah and the beach. Chad had been asking to go back to the beach for some time.

I had set up appointments for my mother, father, Chad and me to go in for massages later in the afternoon of their arrival. I thought that my parents could use the relaxation after their day of travel and Chad enjoyed massages. Rachael did not get an appointment as she was not fond of massages. It was a fun adventure for all of us. My father had never had a massage before, my mother was skeptical as she had had one in the past but it was not a good massage. It was a fun thing for the four of us to do together.

There was a mutual understanding that seemed to create a bond between my mother and Chad. They were both now pretty much confined to wheelchairs and the need of assistance from others to do some of life's functions. It was good to hear Chad voice to his grandmother his feelings he was having about being confined and dependant on others. It seemed to comfort him in some way that he had someone to talk to that understood firsthand his frustration. He felt refreshed and was bright eyed. A visit from his grandparents was just what he needed.

Saturday morning I noticed Chad's face and neck seemed to be swollen. Upon inquiring of it he said he was fine. I voiced my concern that perhaps he should go to the clinic and just have the doctor check him over since we were going to be going out of town. He voiced his concern of perhaps not getting to go on our little trip to Savannah to see his brother and the ocean if he went to the doctor. I reinforced that his health was more important. Reluctantly he agreed. By past experience, he knew that if he saw the doctor for something other than a routine clinic visit that he usually got put into the hospital.

Rachael took him to the clinic to be checked over by the doctor. I soon received a phone call from her to let me know that Chad was having fluid build up around his heart and lungs again. He was going to have to be admitted to the hospital once again. Chad was very upset but knew it was what was best for him.

Upon admission to the bone marrow transplant unit he was settled in and then a procedure was done to drain the fluid. Much fluid was drained from Chad's chest area and he was placed on oxygen and intravenous fluids with antibiotics.

That evening I took my mother and father to the hospital to see him. He was apologetic for messing up the trip to Savannah and insisted that we go anyway. My mother was going to stay with him but he insisted that they still make the trip because it was a place they needed to see. I agreed that it was a trip that could be canceled. He insisted that the trip be made even if he could not go.

The following day was the Little Miss beauty pageant that we had all looked forward to with anticipation. We all felt bad that Chad would not be there to see it with us. We promised to take pictures and a video for him to watch. The pageant was hard on Kiersten. There was much waiting around that made all of the little girls restless. When Kiersten was ready to go on stage a woman accidentally stepped on her hand so she was not in any mood to be on stage. She did get a trophy, a rose, and a certificate and I purchased her tiara crown for her. This was something that I would not recommend any little girl going through until she was much older.

After the pageant Rachael took the pictures and video up to the hospital to let Chad see them. Once again that afternoon I took my parents up to visit him. He once again insisted on us making our trip to Savannah. Chad had never been a selfish person and always considered others feelings. We all finally agreed when he stressed that his grandparents needed to see Shawn while they were here and that we would only be there for two days. I suggested to Rachael that I take Kiersten with us so that she could spend a little more time with Chad at the hospital and not have to worry about finding a sitter. She had already put in for those days off of work so it would be nice for them to spend some alone time. She agreed.

The following morning my parents, Kiersten and I left for our trip to Savannah. We arrived at our hotel on Hutchinson Island where Shawn had acquired top floor rooms with balcony views of the river and overlooking the historical district of Savannah for us. We visited with Shawn and Cathy, went to the beach, rode the ferry across to River Street and toured the town.

Kiersten loved being on the balcony and watching the boats and ships go past. I knew she was going to be a water baby like her daddy and be a beach babe like her grandma and Great Aunt Tina. Chad loved anything that evolved around the water. One of the things he said he was considering after getting well was working for the Coast Guard as a scuba diving rescuer. Again he was thinking of what he could do to help other people in his time of illness.

I called Rachael daily to check on Chad's condition while we were gone. He seemed to be holding steady with very slow recovery. The trip was wonderful but it was good to return back to Atlanta to be near Chad once again.

All too soon it was time for my parents to return to Kansas. We stopped at the hospital so they could say their farewell to Chad. After visiting a short time, my mother and Chad looked at each other straight in the eyes. Softly she said, "I love you, Chad." And Chad replied, "I love you too, Granny." Both had tears in their eyes.

From the hospital we went directly to the airport so they could catch their flight. We said our difficult goodbyes at the airport and I returned to the hospital.

Over the next couple of days I felt as if I was getting a sinus infection or that spring allergies were starting up. Not knowing for sure which it was I called for a doctor's appointment. It took two days before I could get in to see a doctor. I was placed on antibiotics due to the situation of Chad as a safety precaution and told that I could return to staying with Chad after twenty-four hours of antibiotics and no fever. I was glad to hear the news. I had been feeling much guilt for not being there by his side while Rachael was working.

I only made stops in to see Chad for short times instead of staying with him for the next couple days. Rachael would spend as much time as she possibly could with Chad during the daytime and her work schedule of the three days I could not stay with him.

At times Rachael would call me at work that Chad had requested something special to eat or drink and he asked if I would stop by the hospital after work to deliver his request. There were evenings that Chad and I would have a midnight snack of food or drink or both before I went on to the house after work. It was a wonderful time for us. I would sit a distance from his bed as not to spread any possible infections to him even after I had been on the antibiotic beyond the twenty-four hours.

The afternoon of March 16th, while at the house with Kiersten, I received a call from Rachael that Chad had taken a turn for the worse and was going to be moved down to the intensive care unit. The doctor said his kidneys seemed to be shutting down and his liver malfunctioning. They also discovered that Chad had also had another blood clot form in his leg.

I wanted to scream and cry out but held my composure. I prepared the diaper bag and placed Kiersten into her car seat and we were on our way to the hospital. I knew things were not good when Rachael told me that Chad was willing and agreed that he needed to be in intensive care. That indicated to me that he was either in a lot of pain or felt very very ill. I hoped that it did not mean that emotionally he was giving up the fight because he was so ill and tired of all of this battle by now. I was also concerned because the memory of Eric going to the ICU played on my mind. I feared that ICU was the end of the line and the end of life.

I knew the whereabouts of the ICU family room because I had inquired of it before when I went to visit Eric's family. I did not know the whereabouts of the unit itself. Stopping at the receptionist desk on the first floor I got directions on how to get to the intensive care unit. Kiersten and I went down to the basement of the hospital and down a long hall to the back of the hospital. I so desperately wanted to see him and had such an abundance of fear running through my veins.

Rachael came out to stay with Kiersten so I could go in to see Chad. Chad seemed to be resting comfortably. We spoke of how he was feeling, what all the doctors were doing and of general conversation. I sat down on a chair that had been placed by his bedside. He wanted to hold my hand. I fought back tears and fear surged through all the veins of my body at the thought of losing him to this battle. He reassured me that he would only be in intensive care for just a little while.

To my surprise it was cleared by the doctor that we could have one person stay with Chad at all times while he was in ICU. I did not face the reality that it was because they did not have much hope for his survival once again. Chad and I spent our time visiting, watching TV and often me sitting at his bedside while we just held hands as he rested. Oftentimes he did not want to visit but just wanted a touch of a hand close by. I would massage his feet and scratch his head whenever he requested and at times on my suggestion. He never turned down the offer as it helped him relax.

Chad did not seem to be improving much but was holding steady. The doctors seemed favorable for his recovery and talked of him improving. We looked forward to the day he would be transported back up to the bone marrow unit and then home.

Chapter 29
March 2005

A Long Hard Road

I walked along a dreary path
All shadowed by big trees
Thinking of all the problems I hath
Shivering in the cool breeze

Self-pity was my partner
Anger and regret walked by my side
Riding on depression and becoming weaker
Into trouble and turmoil I did collide

There are shadows and strange sounds
Rocks to climb and ruts to fall
There were big things that were abound
And small things that would crawl
Upon something I tripped and fell
Something small yet oh so big to be
As it hit my ears it rang out like a bell
It opened my eyes to let me see

It was a simple book that I found
Covered with dust and with delicate pages
But it was all golden bound
To set me free from all my cages
Now I walk a paved path
With sunlight shining through the trees

DEBBI HUFF

Thinking of all the blessings I hath
Soaking up the warm breeze

Love is now my partner
Joy and sharing walk by my side
Riding on prayers to make me stronger
To handle trouble or turmoil that may collide

HOLDING ON FOR DEAR LIFE

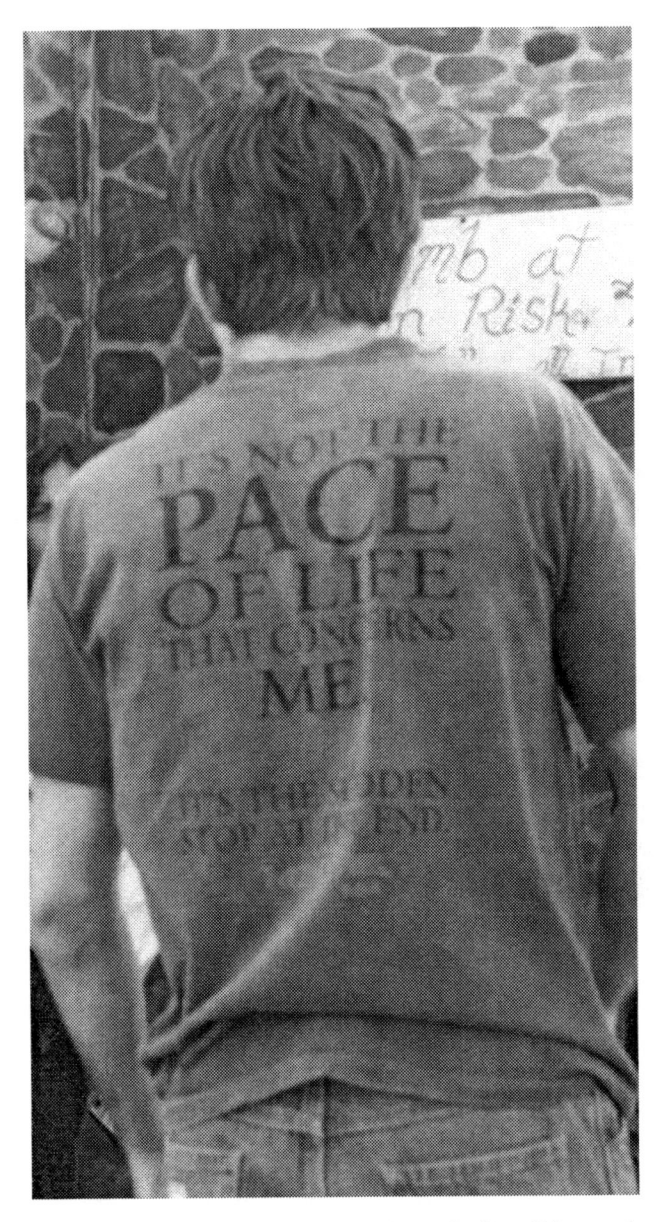

Chad Wore This Shirt a Few Years Before Diagnosis
It Reads: It's Not the Pace of Life That Concerns Me
It's the Sudden Stop at the End

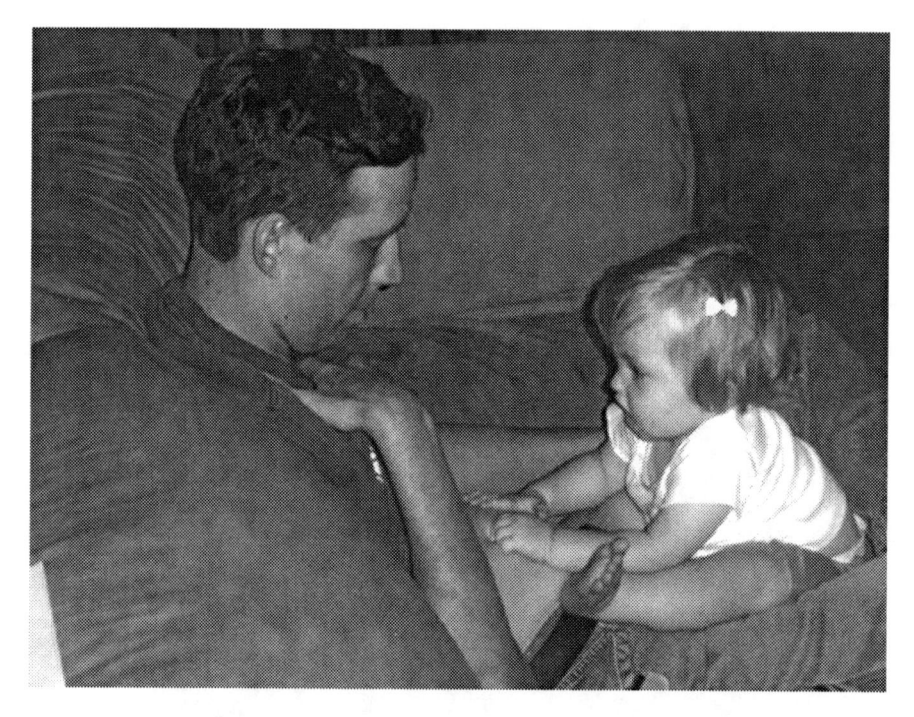

Kiersten Discovering Daddy Has a Belly Button Too

Rachael and I were taking turns staying by Chad's side. Rachael had come up to the hospital to bring Kiersten to me and stay the night on March 18th. For some reason I felt restless and was reluctant to leave the hospital. Yet a good night's sleep in a bed did seem inviting from sleeping in the chair. It also meant I would get a chance to spend a little more time with my granddaughter. I took Kiersten and drove to the house. I knew that with Rachael at his bedside, Chad would be well cared for and have companionship. Before leaving his side I kissed him gently on the forehead and told him I loved him.

Once at the house I settled Kiersten and me in for the evening. I prepared our evening meal and after eating we played for a little while. Soon it was her bedtime.

Kiersten seemed stressed to me for a sixteen-month-old child. She was fussier than usual about going to bed that evening. Rachael had a special music CD that she always played for Kiersten's bedtime. Winnie the Pooh was one of Chad's favorite characters as a child and we sang the Winnie the Pooh song on occasion. When that song came on Kiersten's bedtime CD I started singing it to her. It was a familiar song that I had known for many years and I still remembered most of the words. As I sang tears started flowing uncontrollably down my cheeks for what appeared to be no apparent reason. I had sung the song to her many times before at bedtime and it never affected me in this way.

I tried several times to place Kiersten down to sleep in her bed. Each time I had her settled in and I would start to walk away from her crib she would begin sobbing again. It was not the normal fussy cry. She seemed to be stressed about something.

As I picked her up she pointed to her closed bedroom door and said, "Da-da" repeatedly. This was the first thing that Kiersten had learned how to say. I opened the bedroom door and stepped into the hallway with her cradled in my arms. She pointed to the end of the hallway towards the living room, repeatedly saying, "Da-da." I proceeded to the living room with her. Once in the living room she stopped crying and settled down snuggling in my arms to my chest.

When Chad was a child I sang a song titled "You Are My Sunshine" to him. This song crossed my mind for some reason. I started singing the song to Kiersten. Again tears welled in my eyes and started streaming down my face until I could hardly continue to get the words out of my mouth. Without thinking I changed the words from "Please don't take my sunshine away" to "God don't take my sunshine away."

At that moment the phone rang. It was Rachael calling to let me know that I needed to come to the hospital as quickly as possible. She gave no explanation and I did not want to ask because I knew it was nothing good.

I threw items for Kiersten into her diaper bag and wrapped a blanket around her as I sped out the door. I knew what was going on without being told. Chad's condition had taken a turn for the worse. I knew Chad had come through some tough times and close calls in the past and felt that he would pull through this time too.

I drove as quickly but safely as I could with Kiersten in the car. I was thankful that there was not much traffic that evening and that I seemed to be getting to the traffic lights in time for most of them to turn green.

It did seem strange to me that all the way to the hospital Kiersten was laughing, talking and clapping her hands as if someone was entertaining her. Usually a car ride that late at night would have put her to sleep just a few blocks from the house. As I pulled the car into the parking stall at the hospital parking lot she became quiet. I placed her in her stroller and grabbed the diaper bag.

Entering the hospital I quickly strolled Kiersten's stroller towards the ICU area. I was met just outside the door of the unit by the hospital's family representative. He took both Kiersten and me through a door to a private family waiting area where Rachael was waiting for us. Things must be worse than just a turn for the worse I thought to myself.

I was then informed that they had performed a "code blue" on Chad and that he was now on a respirator. For a second it felt like my own heart had stopped beating. I plopped down in a chair almost in shock. I was glad to not be holding Kiersten at the time for fear I would have dropped her to the floor. My legs became weak as I sat down.

When the turn of events happened Rachael had stepped out of Chad's room only long enough to go to the ICU family room and put on some comfortable clothes for her night's stay at his bedside and brush her teeth. Before she could return the family representative and hospital chaplin came to get her. I thought of how it was like Chad to wait until there was no one with him in hopes to ease any emotional pain they may feel.

Rachael called her aunt to come from Warner Robins, Georgia, and get Kiersten so that both of us could stay at the hospital by Chad's bedside. She graciously came to our side and helped. We made the necessary calls to family. Shawn and Cathy would be arriving in the early morning hours and Chad's father and his wife would arrive in the afternoon. Tina would be arriving that afternoon also.

After what seemed like an eternal wait we were finally told we could go in and be with Chad. Rachael and I were both allowed to stay in the room with Chad together. Chad was being kept partially sedated but was able to wake when aroused. Rachael and I stayed constantly at his bedside and tried to keep him as comfortable as possible. Rachael taped pictures of Kiersten on the bedrails of both sides of his bed so he could see them no matter which side he was lying on. There was hope that this would give him added incentive to fight to live.

In the back of my mind I wondered if Chad knew that death may be approaching. I thought of his picture on his website where the guy is flipping off death (the grim reaper) with his middle finger. I wondered if he was prepared to die or if he wanted to be rescued. His battle had been so long and so hard over the past several years. I knew he was tired of it all. I recalled the times he had asked me to tell them to stop all the treatments and just let him die. Was he welcoming the possibility of having all this over with? I was afraid to ask. I was afraid of the answer I may receive.

Mid morning we were asked to leave the unit so that they could bathe Chad and change his bedding. Rachael and I went to the ICU family waiting area to try and rest a little while we waited for permission to return to Chad's bedside and the arrival of family. Shawn and Cathy were the first to arrive. I filled them in on the event's details. Shawn's eyes filled up with tears and he asked how soon he could go see his brother. Chad's father and his wife arrived next and then Tina.

When we were finally allowed to return back into Chad's room the first to visit was Shawn. Chad attempted to communicate with Shawn but with much difficulty. Shawn's visit was short as he could not stand to see the pain and condition his brother was in. He did not want his only brother to see him weeping. His heart was breaking and he was an emotionally wreak.

Next to visit were Chad's father and his wife. Chad aroused and tried talking to them also. He was weak and tired but let them know he was glad to see them.

When Tina arrived later that afternoon, I took her into Chad's room to see him. I woke him to tell him that his Aunt Tina was there. He looked into her eyes and raised his arms for her to give him a hug. She reciprocated with a hug and a kiss to his cheek. He reached out and held her hand. A most heartwarming and touching moment that made a precious, priceless memory. He was letting Tina know how special and important to him she was in his life. He was so very grateful that she came.

Later that evening I called my friend in Oklahoma that had been giving me comfort with his readings over the course of Chad's illness. After informing him what had happened, he informed me that Chad would be going home in a week and be feeling much better. I was amazed and relieved. Another miracle was on its way.

During the week to follow we took turns staying with Chad in his room and caring for Kiersten after Rachael's aunt returned home. We rotated the times we stayed in the family ICU waiting area, at the house taking care of Kiersten or at Chad's bedside.

For three days there was a large family that basically "moved" into the family room and took up all the space. There was literally nowhere to sit or sleep. Sometimes we had to sleep in a hallway waiting area in a chair to get any rest. The hospital policy was to limit the number of family members staying at night in the family room but it was not enforced. A call to the office assured us that only three family members per patient were allowed to stay over. This still did not help enforce the rule.

Chad remained on the respirator but it was only assisting his breathing occasionally now. He was placed on a dialysis machine to filter impurities from his blood since his kidneys were still not functioning to capacity. He remained on a blood thinner medication to try and eliminate the blood clot from his leg. There were numerous intravenous bags that were at various times from his IV poles that were filled with medications of various sorts.

I spoke to a gentleman during the first part of that week that had his wife also in intensive care. He stated to me that she had gotten a sepsis infection and there was little hope left for her. Fear prompted me to try and observe all who entered Chad's room to see that they gowned and washed their hands before entering.

Chad had been complaining about abdominal pain to me. I voiced this to the doctor who upon exam could not discover any problem. I requested a heat pack for his abdomen and that seemed to give him some relief. If his stomach was touched he would cringe showing his discomfort. Chad was unable to eat normally so his stomach was staying empty. I questioned if this was causing some of the discomfort since he had stomach problems previously due to stress. A feeding tube was once again placed into his stomach so that he would receive nutrition, once again to his dismay.

As the days passed the respiratory doctor stated that she thought he could come off the respirator any day. The infectious disease control doctor stated he thought Chad had sepsis (an infection of the blood) like what he had gotten when he was going through chemotherapy treatments at the beginning of this battle. He had won a battle against sepsis previously but was stronger then. I knew this to be a serious type of infection. His heart doctor said his heart was remaining strong.

Only Chad's oncologist doctor approached me with a straightforward attitude. He informed me that Chad was seriously ill and that he was not sure he was going to be able to survive this time. I reminded him that Chad had surprised us before and perhaps he had another miracle for us. But in my heart I did not totally convince myself with my own words.

Due to poor circulation, perhaps from the blood clot, Chad's feet started turning purple. Because of this, medications were changed and treatments started to increase his circulation. He was also placed under a warming blanket. Chad had been under the cooling and warming blankets in the past and he did not like the blanket. He did not like the respirator tube or the feeding tube. He hated the discomfort of a hospital bed. He did not like having the respirator tube down his throat. We had to watch him closely so that he would not pull anything out. Wrist restraints were placed on Chad and he was strapped to the bed.

I knew he was not resting comfortably and would try to position him as well as possible. Chad would look up at me with sad puppy eyes that told me he wanted all this off and out of him. It broke my heart. I wanted him to be rid of the pain and discomfort but I knew it was what was keeping him alive to try and fight off the illness and survive. I would comfort him with touch and words and kiss his forehead.

After getting permission from the doctor, I would rub Chad's feet gently and scratch his head to try and relax him. I would hold his hand frequently or request to have him turned or pulled up in the bed to try and keep him comfortable. I knew his complaints from the past about the beds of the hospital and the discomfort it caused in his hips and lower back. Rachael spoke with the doctor about this. The doctor ordered a new thicker mattress be placed on Chad's bed for him.

As the week progressed Chad seemed to be stable, however, still critical. The infectious disease control specialist stopped me outside Chad's room door. He approached me regarding the sepsis that was one of Chad's biggest struggles to overcome at this time. He asked me about starting him on an antibiotic. It was the antibiotic that had caused him respiratory problems while he had gotten chemotherapy treatments. However, when he had sepsis in the bone marrow transplant unit they had tried it and it worked. The doctor explained that Chad's system was different at that time since the bone marrow transplant. He tolerated it well then. He reinforced to me that he knew of no other antibiotic to give Chad to fight off the sepsis infection. He reminded me that it had worked the last time they used it and wanted to try it again.

Tina and I talked of her returning home so that she could spend the upcoming Easter holiday with her family. I totally understood and we checked on flights for her to depart on Wednesday, March 23rd, on a morning flight. Chad's father and his wife had made arrangements for their return flight to their home in the Midwest for Thursday, March 24th. Shawn and Cathy had returned home just a couple days before as they had to return to work.

Rachael and I would soon be left alone again to be Chad's support group. We were looking at a slow but progressive road to recovery in our minds.

Chapter 30

Who Has the Right

Who will be there to pick up the pieces
Who has control to say when it ceases
Who will catch you when you fall
Can anyone hear your weak call?

Nothing lasts forever they say
Everything changes day to day
Who has the authority to do this
To take away your glory and bliss?

Who has the right to say when you are through
Who was it that always knew
Was there a clue we missed somewhere
When the pain was too much to bear?

When your heart and your mind are at war
And you do not know what is right anymore
Who can say what is right or wrong
Or where your life does belong?

Who has the right to decide for you
That it is over and done, shades of gray and blue
Who picks up the pieces in the end
When God, for you, an angel does send?

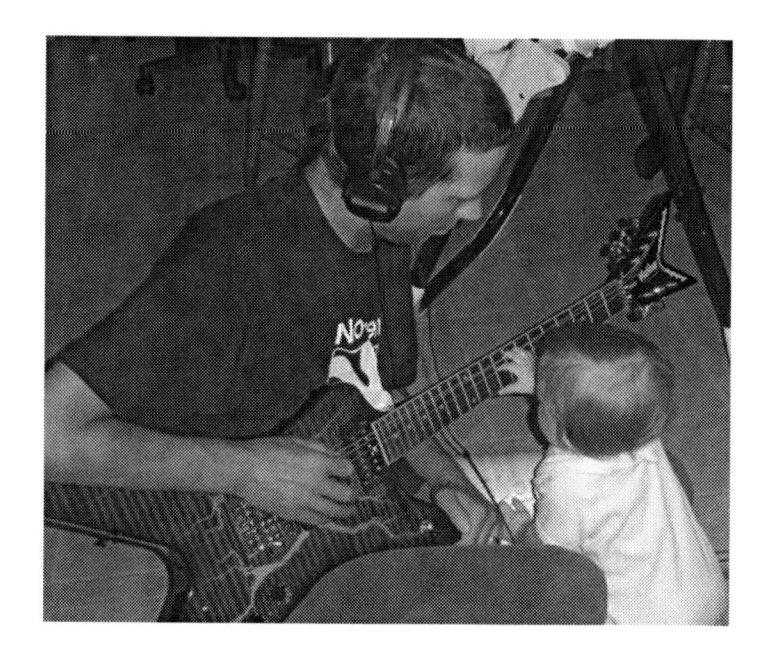

Daddy Shows Kiersten How to Play the Guitar

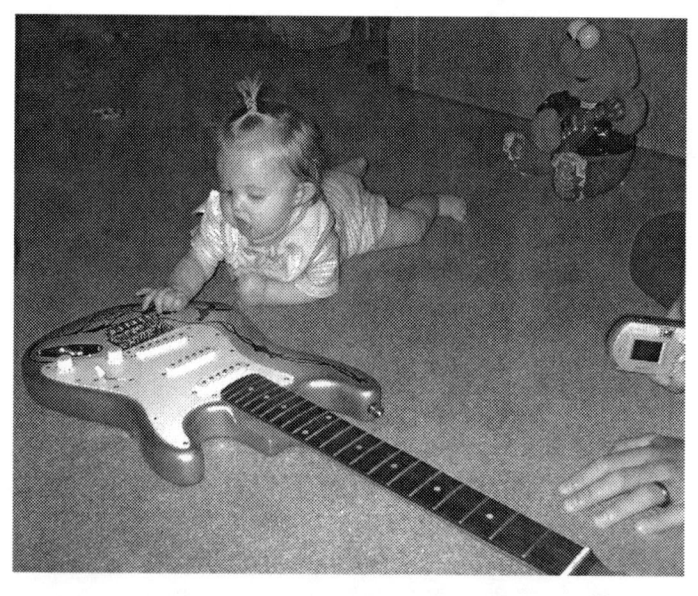

Kiersten with Her Guitar That Mommy and Daddy Had Painted Special for Her for Her Birthday

Rachael stayed with Chad Wednesday afternoon while I took Tina to the airport. It was difficult for me to have her go but I knew and understood why she must. Chad was holding stable and recovery did seem possible now.

Upon returning to the hospital I prepared to stay for the evening so that Chad's father and his wife could go to the house with Rachael. They needed to pack for their return flight the following day.

After their departure from the hospital I positioned a chair directly beside Chad's bed and settled into it. I made acknowledgements to Chad that I was there and reassured him I was there for the night. I sat beside my son's hospital bed in the Intensive Care Unit to comfort him and hold his hand, scratch his head or whatever I could do to help him be more comfortable.

At night it was a dark room located in back of the basement floor of the hospital. I thought of how it seemed like such a cold place with a solid pastel painted cement wall behind his bed and also at the opposite end for his view. On the outer wall were small windows at the top of the wall that let in very little and dingy light. The entry door to the room had a glassed anteroom where once again we scrubbed and adorned gown and shoe covers. Next to the anteroom the glass wall continued with blinds that were kept shut most of the time. On the other side of the glass wall was where the nurses' station was located. This reality was the grim reminder that the end, at any time through any of this, was ever possibly near.

I fought back tears as I sat in silence, except for the sounds of the machines attached to Chad. There was the continuous clicking of the three IV machines regulating medication from the IV bags, there was the hum of the dialysis machine, the click and breathing sounds of the respirator, the subtle sound of air from the oxygen and an occasional "ding" sound from the other side of the glass wall when someone was calling for help. My body shuddered as I thought to myself how this room seemed like one large cement grave that was already mostly underground and how it was such a sad place for anyone to have to be to die. I hated myself for having such horrible thoughts.

The only two things I could point to that brightened up the room was the pictures of my son's sixteen-month-old daughter taped to the bedrails for his viewing. And seeing Chad as he seemed to be resting comfortably as I felt the warmth of holding his hand. I thought of how deeply Chad's love for his daughter was. She seemed to be the reason he was trying so hard to win this battle. His joy and reason for life was in the eyes of Kiersten.

He still had a respirator on to assist him with his breathing, a dialysis machine connected to him to help filter impurities out of his body, the heating blanket that had been placed over him to try and keep his body temperature up to normal, a finger attachment to monitor his vital signs, a machine to observe his heart rate, an oxygen tube in his nose, a catheter to drain any urine, two IV poles with several bags on both, along with various other medical equipment in the room.

Since Chad was being kept partially sedated our conversation was at a minimum that evening. I kept watch, stopping to observe him frequently and to listen so if one of the machines made any different sound than the usual. I continued frequently watching the monitor to see that all vital signs were staying normal. All seemed to be going well and Chad seemed to be resting comfortably.

I was trying to read a magazine to distract my thoughts. I so hoped that it would help me to not dwell on the possible outcome of this situation. I was feeling the loss of my support group since Shawn, Cathy and Tina were now gone. It was difficult as my mind wanted to run rampant with negative thoughts. I prayed to God to give me more faith and strength that I desperately needed at that moment. Somehow in my heart and deep in the pit of my stomach I felt that the battle was coming close to an end. I literally hated myself for thinking and feeling such a horrible thing.

I looked at Chad having to lie in that hospital bed and knew he was not happy. He could not turn himself and could not even move his arms with them tied down.

I recalled that event vividly. As Chad started to get restless two nurses entered the room with straps. Painfully I watched as the nurses placed these straps on his wrists and tied them to the bed frame to keep him from pulling out any of the tubes. Tears welled in my eyes to see Chad's wrists strapped to a bed as I had seen in movies about crazy people in an asylum. He was far from crazy and just wanted to go home.

I so desperately wished that he did not have the respirator on so that we could talk and have a heart-to-heart conversation. A son-to-mother talk. I needed in my heart to know what he was feeling and what he was thinking.

I continually felt ill and tense as I sat by his bedside recalling the words he spoke to me four years ago, "Mom, I don't want to die." I recalled his chemotherapy doctor telling me, "We lose more patients from being neutropenic than from the cancer itself." I wondered if that also applied to losing a patient due to all the medications and treatments Chad had been through. After all, he was in remission right now.

I also recalled the words the doctor had spoken to me just one morning ago, "I don't know if he can pull through this one; he is very very ill." I recalled my response of reminding the doctor that Chad had seen tough times before when the doctors said he was not going to make it through. Chad had shown us miracles in the past but for some awful uneasy feeling I was not sure that it would happen again this time. I searched for my inner strength of my faith.

Late that afternoon as I was sitting there I noticed on one of the monitors that Chad's blood pressure seemed to be steadily dropping. I stepped to his bedside and aroused him. In doing so his blood pressure immediately went back up within normal range and he responded to me. I told him I loved him and kissed his forehead as I touched his hand.

Once again I settled back into my chair that was placed beside his bed. I think somehow I knew that things were coming to an end. I had seen the signs of death so many times with working in the hospital and nursing home setting. I knew there were some things that once started could not be reversed as far as I was aware. Yet I wanted to ignore that this could be happening to my son. The spark of hope seemed to be dimming as my heart seemed to feel heavier.

I was well aware of the pain and suffering Chad had already dealt with and was now dealing with. It caused my heart to ache until it felt like it was going to explode. I knew that Chad would not be happy to be in this condition. I wanted relief for him from all this but not at the expense of it costing him his life. There was a strange pang of guilt that went through my body. It was as if I knew he needed relief from all his trials he had been going through and that there was really only one way for him to reach peace and absence from the pain he was feeling. I then became angry with myself for having such thoughts in my mind.

Evening had been well under way and the late night was closing in upon us. I had been doing final edits on a manuscript titled, "Loving a Married Man, That Is Not Your Husband" for my editor to keep my mind occupied and meet the demands of the deadline. I was becoming very sleepy. Chad seemed to be resting well and his vital signs had been staying normal ever since the late afternoon blood pressure drop.

A nurse came in to check on the dialysis machine and stated that it seemed to be blocked. She stepped out and returned with a new container to place on it. She stated that it would take her a little while to get it replaced and do a few other things that needed to be done.

I informed the nurse that I was going to step out to go to the restroom and get some coffee and I would be back in a short time. As usual I made sure they had my cell phone number if they needed me before my return.

I went to the ICU family waiting area. The room once again was full of people everywhere. I decided to go to the basement coffee machine to get some coffee. I got my coffee and stepped outside the hospital door for about ten minutes for a breath of air. I then returned inside to start my walk down the long corridor to the ICU area. I had been gone about fifteen or twenty minutes total.

As I was almost to the doors of the Intensive Care Unit I heard over the intercom "CODE BLUE ICU. CODE BLUE ICU." My gut and heart wrenched and I knew as I picked up the intercom phone to request entering the unit that it was Chad that was being coded. Somewhere very deep in my heart I had known that his battle was coming to an end but my mind did not want to conceive the idea. As I called to the nurses' station to request entrance into the unit, I was told that someone would be out to talk to me. One of the nurses that knew me well by now from the bone marrow transplant unit in the hospital stepped out to the hall to confirm my suspicion that it was Chad that was being coded.

I was numb. I sat down in a chair that was in the hallway. I stared straight ahead as my mind and body went numb. I wanted to pray for Chad to be revived yet I seemed to have an inner voice telling me to let him go. After a few moments of silence my first thought was to call Rachael. I did so and told her that they had coded Chad again and to come as quickly as possible. I was then taken once again to the dreaded private family waiting area where I had found Rachael sitting only a week before.

The hospital chaplain arrived to sit with me. I impatiently waited for news of Chad. I wanted to let them allow me to be at his bedside no matter what they were doing at that moment. I wanted to see him, I wanted to be at his side, and I wanted him to know I was there and he was not alone and I wanted to tell him I loved him very, very much. I wanted Chad to surprise them all and be well instantly. I then wondered what Chad was feeling and thinking or if he had any concept to what was happening.

I was glad to have someone there with me but wished for someone that I knew to be there. I also wanted to be left alone. The chaplain and I prayed together but I only heard words. Upon completing the prayer the chaplain left from the room. Perhaps he was confused by emotionless blankness. My mind was as if it had shut down and my body was feeling nothing. No anger, fear, rage, sadness, pain, love; no nothing. I felt I should be sobbing and screaming but that would not surface either. Silent tears just continually rolled down my cheeks as I felt that I had just died also.

Again over the intercom I heard, "CODE BLUE ICU. CODE BLUE ICU." The nurse entered to tell me it was Chad again. I did not need to be told this because I somehow already knew. I could feel some anger surfacing because I felt that the hospital staff was causing him to die because they must not be doing all they could do. I questioned if the nurse I had left in the room was still there when this happened.

All at once my bottom lip started to quiver and emotions started to return. My heart felt as it literally was being torn into shreds, tears rolled down from my eyes out of control. I felt nauseated and angered. I was mad at God. Why after all this struggle and so close to returning back to a normal life was God taking Chad away now? I asked this from deep in my heart. It made no sense. Why did he have to go through such suffering and pain if God was going to take him anyway? I did not want him to be suffering but why not recovery instead of death? Why could it not have been me in his place? He had his entire life before him as a husband and father and the ability to make a good career for himself. And here I sit with no mate in my life and not sure what my purpose on earth was anymore. I wished I had stayed numb so I would not have to feel this.

The chaplain had been trying to say comforting words that I did not want to hear. I did not want to hear that God has a set time for each of us to return home to Him. I did not want to hear his seemingly empty words of comfort that fell upon my ears at that point in time. Nothing he said right now was going to comfort me. What happened to ask and you shall receive? The Bible said to ask in His name and in believing it shall be yours? It had worked before and why was it not working now? My faith and trust in God were on the verge of distinction.

The hospital chaplain had come in to sit with me again after the second code blue was announced and was talking to me. I was not hearing what words he was saying but remember that we prayed again. I turned the prayer off in my mind when he started talking of Chad going to Heaven and being with God. He spoke of God's will and Chad in a better place. I was sure that God would accept Chad into Heaven if the medical staff would not save him. But, I did not want to hear of Chad leaving us; that would mean he would die.

That was not the prayer I wanted to pray. I wanted God to let Chad live, let him live to be an old man. I wanted this to all be one of Chad's pranks that he liked to play. I wanted my baby alive and well. I remember thinking that I wished Rachael was already there with me. I felt so alone in a busy, senseless place, with people around me that I did not know and felt that a part of me was slowly dying as my heart seemed to hurt so badly that I did not know if I could withstand it.

The emergency room doctor came into the little room where I was sitting. He told me that the only way Chad's heart would keep beating was when they gave him medication to make it do so and as soon as they stopped giving it to him his heart would again stop. He wanted to know what I wanted them to do. I told him that Rachael was on her way and she could help make the decision. He said there was no time left and what did I want them to do? I asked what the choices were. He said there were none. He said they could not continually keep giving the medication to Chad to keep his heart beating. I wondered why the doctor even had come in and asked me. I thought this very cruel to ask me something that could not be done.

I remembered that Chad had signed a living will and recalled the pain and suffering he had already been through. I remembered the sadness in his eyes as he had looked at me a short time ago as if to say he was tired of all this and wanted it all to stop.

"Is there anything else you can do?" I asked the emergency room doctor.

"I will see," said the doctor and then he left to go be at Chad's side. I wanted to jump up out of my chair and follow him. I thought perhaps if Chad heard my voice it would bring him back to life.

Ten minutes later the nurse came back into the family room to tell me that Chad has passed on and they were going to stop trying to bring him back. She said they had done all they could do but nothing was working now to bring him back.

I was not sure how I was going to tell Rachael upon her arrival. Five minutes later she came through the door with Kiersten in her stroller and Chad's father and his wife right behind her. There was sheer panic and fear on Rachael's face. She looked as though she was on the verge of breaking down. My heart went out to her as I searched quickly in my mind of what to say.

I looked down at Kiersten and tears rolled down my eyes. I had to just tell Rachael straight out that her husband and Kiersten's father was no longer with us. I just stated the fact that they had coded him twice and could not save him. I did not know how else to put it. Rachael stood in disbelief. I picked up Kiersten to hold her close. Our gift from Chad that he left for us as a gift of his great love I cuddled in my arms as new tears streamed from my eyes.

The wait to see Chad seemed like long hours. I first tried to contact Shawn but got no answer. Next I called my parents and then Jeremy. I tried to contact

Tina but got no answer. I do not remember whom else I contacted. Rachael's and Chad's fathers had also been on their phones contacting other family members. It was around three in the morning by then and my mind and body was weak and numb. This all seemed to be a bad dream that we could not wake up from.

Then came the ultimate stab in the heart that caused reality to slap us in the face. We were asked, "What do you want us to do with the body?"

In my mind I wanted to scream, "Bring him back!" Rachael was the levelheaded one and asked them to hold his body at the hospital and we would let them know what funeral home to send him to later that day.

I recalled in the Bible how Jesus cried when he heard his friend had died. However, He brought His friend back to life. Why would he not do that for Chad? What happened to all the promises from the Bible? A year after Chad's death, it was brought to my attention that the reason Jesus cried was because He had to take his friend out of Heaven and bring him back to earth. Chad too was now in a peaceful, happy place.

Like the friend of Jesus, Chad had to go through death twice to get through Heaven's door. I think the delay was because he knew that we did not want him to leave. Yet I wonder if it was because he wanted to tell us something but was never able to because of the respirator and so he just gave up. Perhaps that is why he kept trying to get me to have them take out the respirator tube. It is something that I will never know until I see him again.

At long last we were allowed to go to the room and see Chad. The hospital staff had removed all the tubes and equipment from Chad's room. The room seemed even more cold and so empty now. They had positioned Chad on his back in the bed and his hair neatly combed. He looked as though he was sleeping peacefully after his long days of pain, restlessness and suffering.

Rachael was allowed to take Kiersten into the room and the five of us stood in tears as Kiersten told her daddy "bye-bye" for the last time. I can only wish that Chad could have seen and held Kiersten in his arms one more time before his death. We all stood in silence and disbelief.

I stood by his bedside and reached out my hand. I wanted to hold his hand as he had wanted me to do so many times in the past few days. Rachael stood beside me holding Kiersten in her arms. We then all took our turns going back into the room individually after that to say our own personal final farewell.

There should never come a time in a mother's life when she stands beside her child in disbelief and agony to say goodbye for the last time, unless it be for her own death. In the dark early morning hours on March 24, 2005, I touched my son's face ever so gently on his cheek. I bent down and kissed him on the forehead and told him I loved him. I silently prayed to God that wherever Chad was that he was able to see and hear me and feel the love I have for him in my heart. I vowed to him that I would help raise Kiersten to be as fine a person as her daddy.

Before leaving the hospital we had to let them know what to do with Chad's body. Rachael requested he be laid to rest in St Louis, Missouri, where she was from. It was where the two of them had been united in marriage and Kiersten had been baptized. Her plans were to move back to St Louis in the near future. It was difficult for me to agree to as I wanted his body close to me so I could go visit him often. Yet in my heart I knew that Chad would want to be close to where Rachael and Kiersten were. He loved his little family as I loved mine. The hospital agreed that they would hold Chad's body until we contacted them as to what funeral home the body was to be delivered to.

Rachael, Kiersten and I returned to the house to try and put pieces of what was left of our lives back in some order in our world of total disarray. Chad's father and his wife stayed at the hospital a short time longer until it was time for them to go to the airport for their departing flight that morning.

My sympathy went out to his father as I knew how I would feel if it were me that was flying miles away after my son had just passed away. It was hard enough just leaving the hospital and being in the same city.

The two of them went over to the bone marrow clinic to tell the staff thank you for the wonderful care Chad had received. Upon their arrival all the staff was in tears at hearing of our great loss, including Chad's doctor. Everyone was feeling the large void emptiness left by a heroic wonderful person. Everyone had come to love and enjoy him.

What were we to do now? Where and how were we going to pick up the pieces of this broken family?

Chapter 31

Wings in Flight

In the middle of the night
You slipped away on wings in flight
Loved by all and hated by none
Living life and searching for fun
A sparkling eye and cheerful smile
Helped keep you strong for awhile

Aches and pains, more than your share
For you life was definitely not fair
The intensities of pain you went through
From where was your strength that you drew?

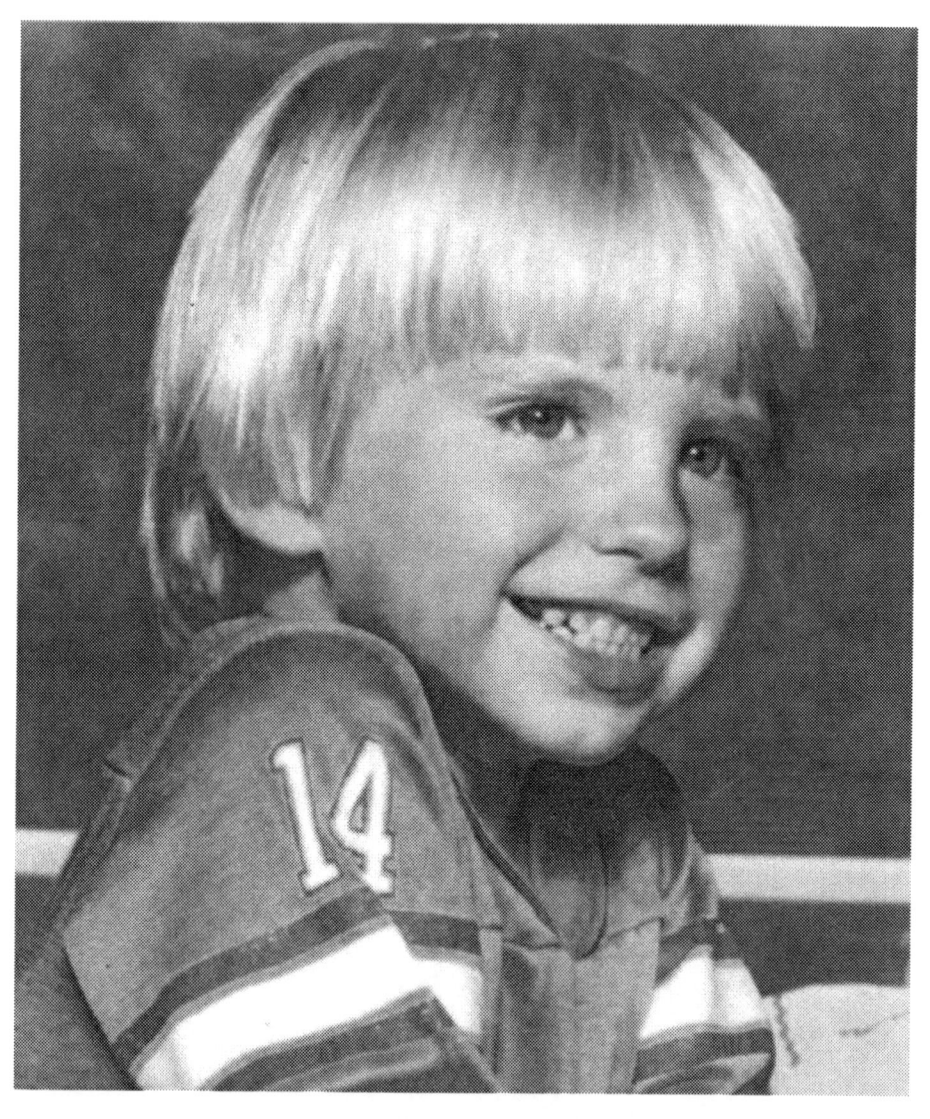

A Beautiful Child of God

After a very short restless sleep I got up and went out to sit on the front porch steps. I wanted to get in my car and drive back to the hospital and sit beside Chad's body. I knew that was not possible. The thought of his body lying in a morgue made me nauseous. I looked up to the trees, flowers, birds and sky and thought of how Chad enjoyed nature so much. I heard cars passing by. This angered me. I thought of how such a great person had just died and so few of the people in this large city even knew it. My world had just come to a stop as I knew it and still nothing seemed to change in the world around me.

Waves of guilt played with my mind as I thought of how Chad was alone when he died. I did not know if I should be angry with myself or that Chad had planned it that way. After all, he waited until Rachael was out of the room the first time he was coded. Then my mind told me that perhaps if I had not left the room he would not have died. Perhaps if I had been there to arouse him like I did earlier when his blood pressure started dropping he would not have died. My mind and heart were in total chaos.

Being the poet that I am I went inside to get paper and pen and returned to my lonely spot where I had been sitting on the porch step. I started writing a poem to Chad to try and ease some of my pain and calm my mind. As I let my feelings of my heart run free through my mind I was amazed at what I was putting down on paper. In my words I wrote:

>Right now my mind and heart remember the pain
>Laughter and tears we shared again and again

The following lines came to my mind almost faster than I could write them down. It was as though I was being told what to write as these words went onto the paper:

>But in time it will fade I know
>As with God I will soon grow
>I will watch my child grow up each day
>And love Rachael in my own way
>My love is all around each of you
>In everything you say and do

I was almost breathless as I read back to myself what I had just written. Tears welled in my saddened eyes. I went inside to tell Rachael and read her the poem. It was as though Chad was comforting us and putting the words into my head that I placed on paper.

If it had not been for Rachael taking charge of making the funeral arrangements I do not know how they would have gotten done. I had no concept of my current world. All I could think of was the emptiness and pain I felt inside. I wanted to just curl up into a ball and disappear. It aggravated me that the world continued on with a normal day when everyone and everything should have been in mourning. Waking to the world after restless sleeps I wanted to just pull the covers up over me and never come out.

During the first week after Chad's death I just went with whatever came along. I was still numb with very little feelings of emotions. I lost the concept of what day and what time it was.

As for Chad's spirit, it did not leave our presence right away. We must have been granted the blessing of his spirit returning after meeting with God, his maker.

Two days after Chad's passing I awoke not wanting to greet the day. I was still lying in bed and kept my eyes closed. I so wanted to talk to Chad so I opened my mind and emptied it of all other thoughts. I had read books on how to talk to angels in the past. I was hoping I would be able to hear Chad. I did. He sounded excited. He told me that there were guitars in Heaven and there were model car race tracks and he was enjoying both with a healthy body that was free of pain. He also informed me that he was there with my grandmother in a nice place. My grandmother is the one that I admired with respect and try to model my life after. I only hope I can be as wonderful a person that she was. I then arose to greet an unwanted day but I could not wait to tell Rachael of my experience.

That same day Kiersten started pointing to the love seat in the living room and then to the bedroom where Chad once slept. While looking at the love seat she spoke two full sentences but we were unable to understand what she was saying. At sixteen months she had just been saying a few simple words. Later that day, while I was gone to the grocery store, Rachael felt strangeness come over her. She informed me that the electricity went off in the house for a short time while she felt this. There were no storms; it was a calm sunshiny day.

That evening I called Shawn to see how he was holding up and he informed me that earlier that evening he was sitting and having a heart-to-heart talk with Chad in his mind. He heard Chad's voice respond to him. It came at a moment that Shawn was thinking about killing himself so that he could be with Chad. With Chad's words, through Shawn's mind, he talked Shawn out of it and reminded him that he was needed to help take care of Rachael and me and to help raise Kiersten.

The following day I contacted Brian, my younger brother, to talk with him. He informed me that he had had a dream two days before Chad's passing but was afraid to call and tell me about it. He had a dream that our grandmother came to him and told him that she was coming to take Chad to Heaven to be with her. There was some comfort in knowing that but it still did not bring Chad back to us.

We had been given a sort of comforting peace in our hearts during our time of pain. However, it still did not help with the events that were to take place over the next two weeks. Decisions had to be made, a trip had to be taken, arrangements had to be made and a burial had to take place.

Chapter 32

Chad's Place

The sunlight shines upon my face
This is such a peaceful place
Colors are vividly rich in hue
The gold, emerald, ruby and sapphire too
Do you feel the worry-free serenity
Freedom from regret, pain and pity?

Oh look, see the fish in the clear sea as glass
Come and let us watch it pass
An abundance of sweet smells to be found
The flowers bloom here all year round
Do you hear the birds singing up above
Oh, see that up there, that covey of dove?

Calming songs in angel voices
As all here in love rejoices
No strangers come into this city
No one is poor so there is no pity
Money has no value here
Isn't it grand to have no fear?

I have lots of new guitars
For fun I race little motorized cars
I scuba dive, surf and swim
And visit with some of my kin
Come and join me in the fun
We will laugh and hug when day is done

HOLDING ON FOR DEAR LIFE

Smiles and laughter are all that is here
Only in gladness do we shed a tear
Oh my, what is that running down your face?
You look like you do not like this place
I forgot this place you cannot yet see
For you have not gone to Heaven yet like me.

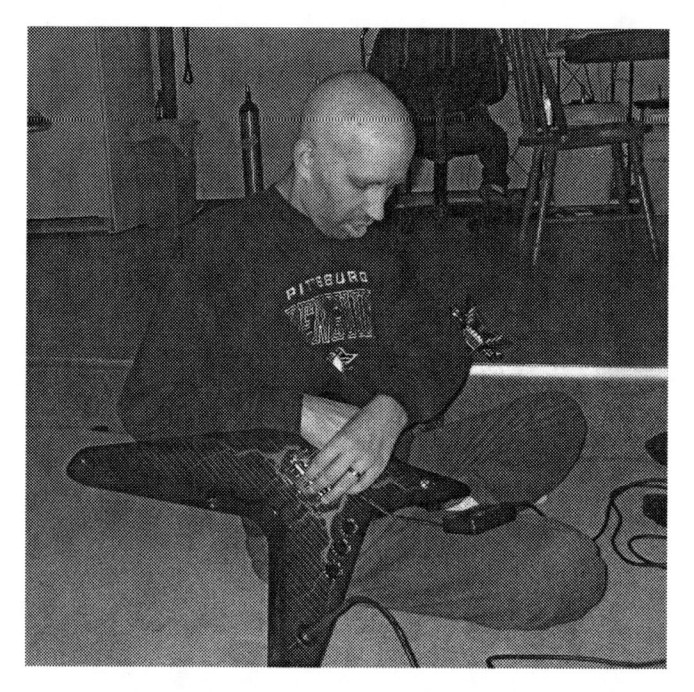

Music Filled His Soul to the Very End of Time

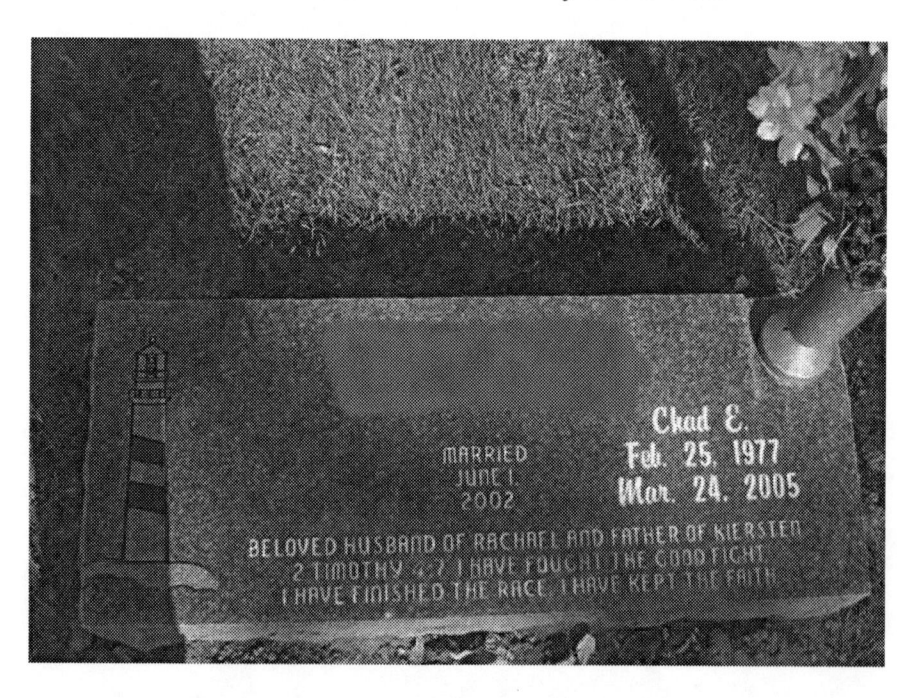

It was decided that the funeral and burial was to be in St Louis, Missouri. Part of me wanted him to be buried in Savannah because he loved the place so. I did not like the idea of him being so far away but understood Rachael's request. She wanted to have him close for her and Kiersten. I also knew in my head and heart that Chad would want to be close to where Rachael and Kiersten were. Rachael still had plans for her and Kiersten to move to St Louis and wanted him close to them. I did want Kiersten to always know of her daddy and how much he loved her. This would be done more easily with him close to her. Rachael's family would then be close to her for support and comfort.

In Chad's honor we decided it would be on April Fool's Day. We knew that Chad would enjoy that since he liked to tease and play harmless pranks.

I was pleased that Chad would get to fly to his final destination. As a young boy he dreamed of being a pilot. I thought this interesting because the first time he flew was when I took the boys to visit my cousin Tony and his family and to see Disneyland in California. As the plane was descending he became nauseated and vomited. Tony lived with his wife and two children up on a mountain. As we drove up the winding road it made Chad feel ill again. Chad and I got out of the car and walked hand in hand up part of the mountain road. The airlines that carried him on his first flight to California now carried him to his final destination in St Louis.

A few months before his passing he told me that one thing he always wanted to do was to sit in the cockpit of an airplane as it flew just to see what it looked like. He never did make it into the cockpit of an airplane but he did get to see what it was like to fly himself!

Shawn, Cathy, Rachael, Kiersten and I drove to St Louis. The plane that carried Chad to St Louis would be arriving about the same time that afternoon as we were to arrive into the city.

Rachael and Kiersten settled into her father's house and Shawn, Cathy and I settled into a hotel. It was hard being apart from Rachael and Kiersten. Rachael had been the strong one. For once in my life I could not keep up my guard and my weakness prevailed. It was difficult to try and keep my mind off my pain with such a heavy heart. I tried to keep my mind off the events that would be following in the next two days. I knew that the following day we would be selecting a casket, flowers, and making funeral arrangements.

The following morning Rachael and I were to meet with the funeral director at the funeral chapel. Her father came to help us and watch Kiersten. I pulled my car into the funeral home parking lot and shut off the engine.

Rachael had not yet arrived. There was a funeral going on and an overwhelming sadness came across me. As I watched the funeral guests I sobbed at the thought that that would be my family tomorrow. I looked forward to family arriving for my much-needed comfort. When Rachael arrived we selected the flowers, casket and other items that were needed. I know there were other things discussed but they were a blur to my mind. I remembered all the times I had tucked Chad into his little bed at night as he grew to be the wonderful man that we were selecting his final pillow to rest his head.

It was discussed as to what Chad would be wearing. Rachael had picked out his maroon shirt and a tie and dark slacks. He always looked so handsome dressed up with his unforgettable smile. She then informed the funeral director that we had a pair of shoes for him to wear. He said we did not need those. Rachael informed him that we did need those. Chad had a pair of multicolored canvas shoes that he was dearly attached to. As they started becoming worn out we searched for two years to find him another pair. We had no success. The funeral director agreed to put them on him. Rachael also gave him Chad's green plaid flannel shirt to place into the casket just before its closing. This was another item that was Chad's favorite to wear as a light jacket.

That afternoon Shawn, Cathy and I went shopping. Shawn did not have a suit and he wanted one to wear. For him it would be a sign of respect for his brother. He did find a very nice suit and looked very handsome. I thought about how he and Chad wore the same size clothes. I thought how Chad would get a chuckle out of his brother wearing a suit but also in his heart he would be very pleased that Shawn wanted to show how much his brother meant to him.

While at the mall I stopped in a jewelry store to browse. The boys always teased me about my "bling-bling." That was what they called my jewelry. To my pleasure and delight I spotted a silver and gold bracelet that was a row of butterflies. The gold trimmed the butterflies and made up their bodies and antennas. The silver was as detailed lace for their wings. I thought of how I had seen the white butterfly in the garden the first evening that Chad had called me when he was diagnosed. Rachael also had told me that her father was going to say something about butterflies at the funeral sermon. There was also a private running joke between Chad, Shawn, and myself about me and a butterfly. This was the perfect piece of jewelry for me. The purchase was made, I put it on and will not take it off unless it breaks or I die. In that event it will be passed on to Kiersten.

The following afternoon was visitation at the funeral chapel. I held up well. I kept myself busy with greeting family and friends and taking care of Kiersten. I was pretending in my mind that it was just a big family get-together and not for a funeral.

Family and friends were gathering in the city of St Louis to pay final respects and farewells. Many drove for long distances and even friends that had not been seen for many years came to say goodbye and show their respect. Chad touched so many lives in such positive ways.

Some of my closest friends and family stayed with us at the same hotel. The night before the funeral we gathered in the dining room/bar of the hotel. Chad's cousins Joshua, Jeremy, Melissa, and Debi were there along with Tina and my brother Danny, Shawn, Cathy and me. I knew that Joshua and Jeremy were feeling the loss like it was a brother, the same as Shawn. I knew that Tina and Danny were feeling the loss like second parents. As we sat at the bar talking, we all voiced the feeling of Chad in our presence and how he would be enjoying us all being together. We were missing him being the life of the party and making everyone laugh.

I told them all the story of Chad and Eric and how they had planned to be drinking a beer together on the porch. As honor to them both we all had a beer and, in our mind, pretended we were there drinking it with them.

Later that evening Debi informed me that her two-year-old daughter, Lacey, pointed to the door inside their hotel room that led to the hallway. Lacey asked her who that man was that was standing there. Debi questioned her as to what the man looked like. She described Chad. It warmed our hearts to know that Chad was still with us, even if only in spirit.

The following morning I placed a call to Lisa to see how soon she was going to be arriving. Sobbing, I told her that I could not do this on my own any longer and needed her there for strength and support as soon as she could get there. She informed me she was on her way.

I moved blankly from task to task in preparing to depart from the hotel to the funeral home. My mind had reached the level of denial and numbness that I never knew existed. Another of my closest friends arrived to stay with me at the hotel, Elaine. She had driven from Oklahoma all by herself and borrowed the money to make the trip. Having family and friends close by my side to guide me was a comfort. I had to literally keep forcing myself to do anything. Somehow I seemed to think that if I did not go to the funeral it could not take place and would not be real.

During the funeral the numbness remained in my heart and my mind. I tried to listen to the sermon but it passed by my deaf ears. I could hear words but nothing was making any sense. I sat on the front church bench and was surrounded by people. Yet I felt so alone in a heartless world. I could not take my eyes off the casket that now held a part of my heart and my son. I remember asking myself why I was not crying hysterically. Had I cried all the tears that were ever in me? Was it that I was so numb that I had no feeling left inside me?

I tried to remind myself that he was now at peace and free of pain. It did not last. My thoughts kept going back to all the joyful things in life that he should be living and to continue doing. I thought of my little boy and the joys that he had given to so many of us sitting in the filled-up church. I thought of Shawn who had lost the only brother he had ever known and how lost he must be feeling. All the fun and shared times they had together were now just memories. I thought of how brave and heroic Chad had been through all his agonizing treatments and procedures.

I remember wondering how Shawn, Rachael, my parents, Tina, Danny, and Jeremy were holding out with their emotions. I thought of how he had told me that he did not want to leave Rachael a bride and a widow in the same year when he was diagnosed. I thought of the sixteen-month-old little girl that would never get to have her daddy there for her.

Now Chad's body lay motionless in the very church where the two of them had exchanged wedding vows and became one in the unity of God. The very church where his little girl was baptized.

Reality came back to me as part of the sermon touched on my ears. The preacher (Rachael's father) spoke of how a caterpillar starts out, spins its cocoon, waits for awhile, and then emerges as a beautiful butterfly. Just as we are as a caterpillar here on earth, spin a cocoon and then with God's graces we are taken to Heaven as a beautiful new butterfly in a new pain-free body.

I continued to manage my composure until the service was over. I sat watching my family slowly pass by the coffin to say their final farewells. Tears began to well in my eyes. When my father pushed my mother up to the casket in her wheelchair is when the first heart wrenching thing called reality began to haunt me again. As I saw my parents begin to cry, my tears ran freely.

When everyone else had been ushered out of the church we were ushered out to the lobby after passing by the open casket. Standing in the lobby I stared through the window to the sanctuary as the picture of my son's casket in front of the alter burned into my brain. As I saw the funeral director approach the coffin, I rushed to get out of the church. I could not stand the thought of the lid to the casket being closed down over Chad. That meant I would never see him again.

From the funeral home we proceeded in caravan style to the cemetery that would be Chad's final resting place. As we were walking from the cars to the gravesite Rachael saw some dog feces on the ground. She had warned several people about it as they walked by. She then ended up stepping in it herself. We all decided it was Chad playing an April Fool's joke on her which made us all smile.

I do not remember what the weather was like. I was not cold and I was not warm. Nausea, headache and sorrow began to overwhelm me as I saw the casket removed and carried by his most beloved friends and family men. As we walked behind the casket my body started to tremble. As they placed the casket onto the stand I wanted to scream; I wanted to run away. Instead I stood fast until we were seated in chairs alongside the casket that was protected by a canopy.

It was not until the final blessing over the casket that I could no longer hold in my emotions. It was as though everything that had been held back by the numbness burst itself inside me, screaming to get out. Through flowing tears I sobbed, "I don't want to be doing this." I did not want to be sitting there with my son about to be buried. I wanted him to be alive and for me to be allowed to be in the casket in his place. My fear of death did not matter anymore.

With assistance of close friends I stood to depart with the guests. I proceeded over to the floral spray that I had gotten for him that had been placed at one end of the casket on a stand. It was made up of red roses and white carnations. There was a large red bow that had a ribbon flowing from it that said "Beloved Son." I selected a red rose with velvety petals that seemed to be the most perfect one of them all. After placing it onto the top of the casket, I kissed the inside of my fingers and placed my hand onto the top of the casket. I paused for a moment as if I had become frozen in time.

As I was being assisted in walking back towards the car my mind relocated itself back to what was going on. I was walking away from my son and leaving him to be buried into the ground. I instantly thought of Shawn and asked where he was. He stepped up beside me from where he had been walking behind me. We placed an arm around each other as we slowly walked away from the site of burial. I recalled what my father had told me many years ago, "I hope I die before any of you kids do." I used to think that was so mean for him to say but now my mind kept repeating, "Your children are not supposed to die before you do."

At that point my mind started telling me that this was all a dream and not really taking place. Perhaps that is what they mean by the body being in shock. I do not know. I do know I was able to stop the tears. Throughout the rest of the day I was almost able to pretend that everything was just a dream. I seemed to have convinced my mind it was, once again, just a big family/friend get-together and tomorrow everything would be back to normal.

Upon arriving back to the church we were welcomed with a noon meal that had been prepared by the ladies of the church. I noticed I had a voice message on my cellular phone. I had received it around ten in the morning, which was the time of the funeral. Upon listening to it I could not make out the male voice or exactly what it was saying. Family and friends had come from all over the states and I could not figure out who it would have been. I will never know who the message was from or what they were saying but in my heart I would like to think it was Chad trying to tell me goodbye, that he loved us, and that all was well with him. I have heard of stranger things that have happened. With him having the respirator in place the last week of his life it was impossible for him to speak with me, which I so desperately wished he could have.

The evening of the funeral Rachael requested that I make a call to my psychic friend in Oklahoma. It lay heavy on Rachael's heart to know if Chad had made it into Heaven and she wanted me to ask him. At first I did not want to because I was mad at him. He had told me that Chad would be going home in a week when I talked to him after the first time Chad had been coded. I felt like he had lied to me just so I would not know he was going to die.

At Rachael's request I did make the call. My friend informed me that Chad got to see the face of the Lord shortly after he passed on. He also informed me that it was an older woman, an older man and a younger man that came to get him. I felt the woman was my grandmother and the older man to be my grandfather. As for the younger man I was not too sure but felt it must have been Eric, the young man that Chad had agreed to sit on the porch with for a beer and teach how to play guitar before his passing. When I informed Rachael of this she too thought it to be Eric because she said she had asked him in thought and prayer to be there for Chad when he passed on. Shawn also voiced that he thought it to be Eric.

Being friends I also felt I could quiz him about telling me that Chad would be going home after the first time he was coded. He asked me, "He did go home, didn't he?" All of a sudden the picture became very clear through the fog. Chad was all better and he did get to go home. It was just not the physical home here on earth that I had been thinking about. He was well and at his final home with God in Heaven.

Since that time there have been fewer and fewer times of feeling Chad's presence. I think that he is still with us in spirit but has become a comfortable feeling. We all still talk to him in our hearts and minds. He will always be alive in our hearts and minds.

I know that time will not let me forget or make things better. I know that my heart will always ache with every holiday, birthday, anniversary, date of death, date of funeral, any day that had any type of special meaning. It aches with anything that is said or that I see or hear that reminds me of my little boy during his lifetime with us.

I have learned that I do not have to forget, that the ache in this mother's heart will never go away and it is okay to cry. I do know that I am learning, over time, how to deal with these feelings and how to handle the emotions better.

I am no longer mad at God and am thankful that Chad is pain free and in a place with other loved ones that have departed this earth before him. I still do not understand why Chad had to go through such a painful trial and why he was selected to leave this earth after such a short time. I do know that when I reach Heaven I will see him again and all my questions will be answered. As my faith is slowly rebuilding I know that Chad will be waiting in Heaven with open arms to receive a hug from me on the day that we are once again living in the same place.

This mother's heart will never be the same. A part of it is missing; a part of it left me on March 24th of the year 2005. This part will never be refilled or replaced until my little family is once again whole. With each ache it remembers that it has been blessed by knowing the true meaning of unconditional love and the value of life lessons learned from her son.

Chapter 33

All Too Soon

Only for a short time I had you to hold
All too soon my arms grow cold
The emptiness I now feel inside
Hurts my heart until I want to hide

You made me laugh, you made me cry
Something new you were always willing to try
Adventure and travel sparked your soul
Enjoying life seemed to be your goal

All too soon you went away
A part of my heart went with you on that day
To continue on without you is hard to do
But I will always remain a mother to you

You have taken that final step
As your soul from earth leapt
The final journey you have made
As into this earth your body was laid

HOLDING ON FOR DEAR LIFE

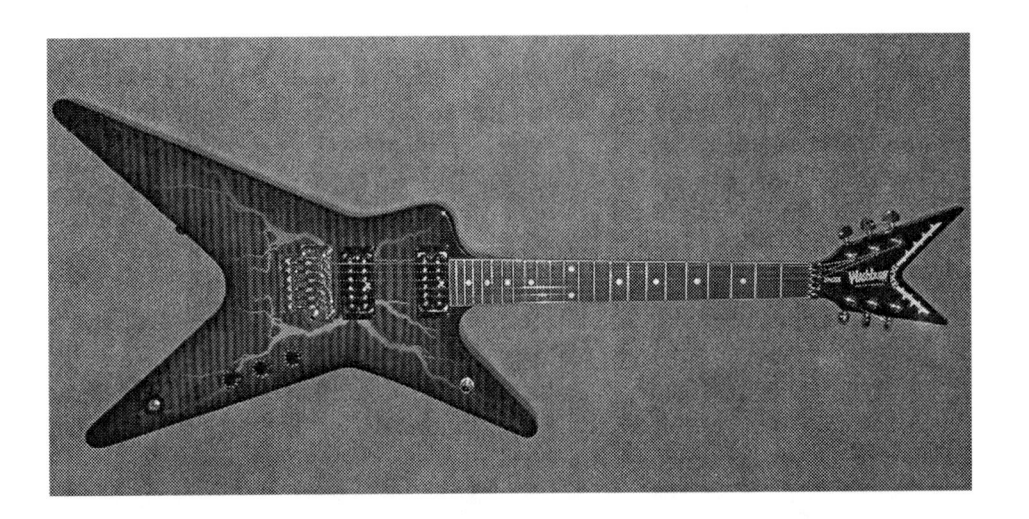

One Guitar Stands in Silence Full of Memories and Love

Chad had gone through four years of what some people would call "hell on earth" for his family. The times when he wanted it all to stop and for us to just let him die, he still continued the fight. To have seen the suffering he went through because he loved us so much and knew how much we loved him was more than any human should have ever had to endure. His suffering was long and hard but he fought the battle hard. Leukemia was his enemy but all the treatments and medications were the army that won the battle.

It is with great honor and pride that Chad's story is told. I know too that others have walked or are walking in similar shoes. My heart goes out to each of them for their battle is sometimes long and the road is very rough with many mountains to move. I look to those who have walked this road and can say that they are survivors and I am joyful for them and their families. At times I wish I could be in their shoes because of a mother's aching heart. Chad was a survivor of leukemia but not of the treatments and medications that were used to try and save him.

Shawn and my lives were blessed by Chad being a part of our little family. Chad blessed me with giving me a daughter by the name of Rachael. We were fortunate to be blessed with four extra years from his time of diagnosis because of the treatments and medications. Our family was blessed by Chad adding Kiersten to it before he departed from it. Many people were blessed with getting to have their life paths cross with Chad's, for he touched everyone's life in a special way that he did meet. To know him was to love him as you will see by the memorial letters to follow.

> *To my beloved husband and partner,*
>
> *I thought I would write a letter to you today, just to be different from all of the other entries.*
>
> *There are so many things to write about one special person. You can't really sum up everything in one page, so many different experiences and journeys in the seven short years we had together. Some say that seven years isn't really that long to be with a person, and of course you haven't known that person as long as their parents. A wise person once said, though, "You don't choose who you are born to, but you do choose the person you are with," so I think that makes the relationship just as strong. So many things shared together with only that one person. So many roads and paths taken in a short amount of time.*

I remember when we met—you came over and never left. I think I fell in love with you that night and that's why I would never leave you until your end. I was angry with God for a while when he took you to Heaven. First he took my mom away, and then you, my husband and Kiersten's daddy. I didn't understand why and what lesson I was supposed to learn from all of this. We were supposed to grow old together and have wheelchair races, along with so many other "supposed to have done things." I felt like it was my fault. Maybe you would have gotten better if I had quit work and stayed home with you all the time, or maybe if I had treated you better somewhere along the way. But then I remember our conversations about how we have to keep going, and someone has to pay the bills and take care of everything. Sometimes I still feel like I treated you wrong and this was God's way of teaching me a lesson, but somewhere in this journey I have come to realize that we really did okay for the circumstances, and God has a plan for each of us, even though we may not see it quite yet.

I remember lying in bed one night, about two days before you passed. I prayed to God asking him to help you, even if it meant you were supposed to be in Heaven. That was the hardest prayer I have ever said, and I guess God decided that this was enough for all of us to bear. I have always believed that God gives us only what he thinks we can handle, and I think that was God's cutoff point for me.

I loved you very much, and will love you always. You made me laugh, even though I tried not to (so not to encourage you!). Luckily, your "retarded" gene, as we jokingly called it, was passed down to you daughter. I see it every day, for example, when she strips down naked to use the potty, just like her daddy.

I think what I really want to tell you in this letter is how much I loved you. I thank God every day for our beautiful daughter and all of the good and bad times we went through. You were a wonderful father in the short time you had with Kiersten. She really loved you, and I hope someday she will be able to tell everyone about her daddy and how brave he was until the end.

You were the bravest person I know. Even in the worst times, you still thought of others, and rarely complained. Your long fight, and defiance towards the doctors amazed everyone, and I was so proud of you for defying their odds so many times.

The hard part about starting this letter was how to close it. I think I will end it with the Bible verse my dad helped me pick out from 2 Timothy 4:7 – "I have fought the good fight. I have finished the race. I have kept the faith." I think this is such a powerful verse because you were a true fighter and you really did finish your battle with leukemia because you were in remission when you passed away. And now a poem to close.

*When your tomorrow starts without me
And awaking, you do not see me
Do not let the sunrise find your eyes
Weeping with tears for me
I truly do not want to have you cry
Because of things we did not say as time passed us by*

*I know that you loved me as much as I loved you
And know that in my heart I am missing you too
When your day starts and beside you I do not stand
Know that an angel came to take me by the hand
And said, God had my place ready in Heaven above
And I could not take along with me the ones I love*

*As I started to depart, tears filled my eye
For so often I had said, I don't want to die
There was so much to live for and yet so much to do
It was so difficult leaving Kiersten and you
I thought of past days, both good and bad
I thought about what we shared and the fun we had*

*If I could have back yesterday just for a little while
I would tell you I love you and good-bye, hoping you would smile
But yet I know that this can never be*

HOLDING ON FOR DEAR LIFE

And tomorrow's emptiness and memories would replace me
When I pondered on things I will miss tomorrow
And think of you, my heart felt such sorrow

But entering through Heaven's gate felt just like home
To see my Father smile at me from his great throne
He said, "This is eternal life, as I promised you
Your life on earth is done and here it starts anew
I never promised tomorrow and today will always last
As each day is peaceful there is no hurting for the past

You have remained trusting, faithful and true
I look beyond the things you weren't supposed to do
It has been forgotten and forgiven, you are now free
Come take my hand and share a pain free life with me
Know when your tomorrow starts without me, we are not apart
Every time you remember me I am right there in your heart

I will love you always.

Love,
Me (Rachael)

I have many fond memories of Chad as I watched him grow from a baby into a man, but the most memorable are when he would sit around the kitchen table with Jeremy, Josh and Shawn and recite movie or TV lines. Or when they were really being creative and made up their own versions of the movies. It was hard to stay in your chair; you would be laughing so hard.

I remember the day Deb called and told me Chad had been diagnosed with AML. I was in shock and disbelief. Then I started the frantic arrangements to get to Atlanta. That would be my first of many. That first trip taught me a lot about Chad. Or should I say Chad taught me a lot about life.

Chad was always brave even though he was scared. I pulled from his bravery to try to help comfort him when he was scared and sick. He would apologize when he would get sick from his treatments, more concerned about the feelings of those around him. We watched a lot of cooking shows even when food made him nauseous and funny movies when he didn't feel like laughing. He was always concerned that I had a good time and didn't get bored.

We went to Hilton Head before he started another round of chemo and was able to spend some fun time at the beach and going out to eat. He loved the beach and we talked about another trip we had taken, to Cancun.

Chad always had such a zest for life. Whether it was riding bikes, skateboards, boogie boards, or just sitting and visiting, he always had funny things to say and was fun to be around.

Chad's great personality, humor, and bravery are what I think of and try to feed off of when I think of Chad. I treasure my memories and they will always be with me.

God be with you, Chad, till I see you again.

Aunt Tina

I'll never forget receiving the phone call when my wife informed me that my cousin Chad had leukemia. I was sitting in the studio in Los Angeles on a Saturday afternoon when the phone rang. My producer and the other band mates tried to console me, but I didn't listen to anything until I talked to Chad and Aunt Debbie. I have to say that Chad, Shawn and Aunt Debbie were the light throughout Chad's fight. Chad and Shawn have always been like brothers to me more than cousins, and my aunt Debbie a surrogate mom.

Chad and I always loved comedy. We would listen to comedy albums every time we were together. One time Chad fell off our swing set laughing at the "Drive-in" skit on our favorite comedy album at that time. More than once we had acted out skits for our parents. He always knew all the new comedians and most of their lines word for word. Chad loved to make you laugh. He would even make jokes at his own expense just to see you smile.

He loved life and everything about it. He loved to meet new people and learn new things. Everyone and everything was important to him. Just like the time when he heard the Ice Cream Man's music coming down the street. He wasn't about to not get his favorite icicle off that truck. So much so that he ran full speed, smack dab into the glass storm door and lit flat on his back. We laughed about that every time we saw each other. He also loved to mess with the dreaded telemarketer. Whenever I talked to him, I would come away with another way to abuse the next telemarketer. Chad never let ANY opportunity go by.

We also enjoyed music together. My dad, brother and I have always played drums. Chad appreciated music to the full extent. He understood it as a musician does but never played an instrument. It was later in his life that he decided to learn how to play guitar. One night in my basement we had our first chance to play together. It was very informal and Chad was a little scared at first, but it ended up being a great experience for everyone there. Pantera was his favorite group. I remember when he called to tell me he won an autographed album off of a web site. Not long after that, he got a "Dimebag" signature guitar from Rachel. He was so proud of that guitar! We always talked of buying guitars, repainting them, and then selling them on the internet.

Then Chad sent me a guitar for their daughter, Kiersten. Our uncle Brian and I painted it and sent it back to them in Georgia. When Joshua, Melissa and I went out to see them I put it together for her (Kiersten is so beautiful and reminds me so much of Chad). Believe it or not, with Chad on the East Coast and me on the West Coast, we recorded a song via the Internet. It is a song that we wrote together called "The Color Blue." "The instrumental version is o.k. But...I think you should stick to the drums," Chad said about my terrible singing. I (and everyone else will agree) don't sing very well. But I wanted to give him an idea of how the lyrics would go. We had a great laugh at my futile attempt. That was Chad. He would tell you what was on his mind.

*The most important thing that stands out for me is the fact that throughout Chad's entire fight with leukemia, **NOT***

ONCE did he complain, expect pity, or special treatment. In fact, it was like pulling teeth out of a hungry lion's mouth just to get him to talk about it. I never pushed the subject for the simple fact that we always had so much fun talking with each other. I didn't want to bring him down by talking about it. I would ask, "How are you doing?" and his reply was always, "All right, how are Debi and Lane?" There were only two times he ever told me (after I asked) he was "tired of it all." Two times in four years! If only we could all be that strong. And speaking of that subject, he was that strong because of the way he was brought up. His mother, my aunt Debbie, should be proud to have raised two children that are so strong. Chad has been a HUGE inspiration in my life. Not a week goes by that I don't think of him...

R.I.P., brother Chad. I love you.

Jeremy

I've known Chad all of his life, since I'm his older cousin by a few years. With this in mind I have a story to share.
One night Chad and I decided to go out. We went to a bar, walked in the door and the bouncer checked our ID's. We were both under age to drink. The bouncer handed my I.D. back and stamped my hand "under age." He then gave Chad his I.D. and told us to go on in. Chad and I go in all calm and cool. When we are out of sight of the bouncer we start to freak out because Chad was able to buy us beer. He was reluctant at first but that wasn't anything that a little persuasion couldn't fix. The kicker was that I had to listen to Chad give me a hard time about my younger cousin had to buy me beer because I wasn't old enough to buy my own.
Chad loved life and was so full of life that he was the type of person you wanted to be around. He was always laughing and joking. No matter what kind of mood you were in, he would at least make you smile. Even when my brother, my wife, and I went to visit him in the hospital, when he didn't

feel good, he was still cracking jokes. I think some of his humor came from all of those Cheech and Chong tapes he used to listen to.

Chad also loved music and playing his guitar. My fondest memory is when my dad, brother, and I took turns playing drums and jamming with Chad while he played his guitar.

Chad was more like a brother than a cousin. I still envy the way he lived life and not let life live him. I truly believe the world was a better place with Chad in it. I can just imagine the excitement he is causing in Heaven. May God bless you all.

*Until we meet again,
Josh*

I can remember the time of a very special summer. I received a phone call from Debbie. I was so excited that they wanted to share a week of their summer vacation with me and my sons. Eddie, Patrick and I loaded up on the motorcycle and headed for a most wonderful vacation.

The day that we arrived, Chad was right there to take charge. He made Eddie and Patrick feel like they were at home. They played and laughed so much it was hard to quiet them all down for bed time. But when they stopped for just a minute they were all out for the night.

Chad was so protective of his little brother Shawn. He always treated his baby brother as if he would break and no one could be too careful around him. I kept teasing him that I was going to take his brother home with me and he was very sure that I was not. You know the big, "NO, Mom!"

I can remember every time I saw Chad and the family, he was always so happy, so positive, he knew what he wanted and achieved most everything he tried. Head strong, sure footed, and enjoyed life to its fullest.

I do know that he was and will always be a blessing to have known. Even though his time on this world was short he touched so many people, so many lives. And as long as he lives in a memory, in a heart, in the eyes of a little girl he is never really gone. Every time I think of him my first thought is that sweet little blond-headed boy with the great big smile welcoming me and my sons into his home with open arms.

He will be truly missed.

Rhonda

Memories of Chad

I met Chad when I was a new nurse on 5 North at Piedmont Hospital. I think it was the summer of 2002. When you are getting report on a patient and you hear "AML" you inwardly cringe because you know that person has a long, rough treatment ahead, and usually not with a great outcome. This was even more difficult because Chad was younger than I was, and that is always a sobering thought. You walk in the room not knowing what to expect, because this person was just diagnosed with a potentially deadly disease.

I walked in the room and made a friend.

I loved Chad instantly. He was hilarious, sarcastic, outgoing, outspoken, and so much fun to take care of. You could sit with him and watch TV. You learned quickly when he liked to have fun and when he wanted you to leave him the hell alone. He's been known to yell at doctors if he didn't like what they had to say or didn't discharge him in a timely manner. He wasn't afraid to challenge you and say "Why are you giving me that cough medication? Won't it MAKE me cough?"

Chad's favorite thing to do to pass time was to scare the student nurses. Every fall and spring we have them on our unit. I've been a student nurse, so I can only imagine how these poor students felt. You are scared to death to be taking care of a real person, much less someone your age with a disease you know nothing about. The student nurse came to me, looking like a deer in headlights, and told me that Chad had lost some hair. I explained to her this was perfectly normal after receiving chemotherapy and Chad knew he would be losing his hair so it was nothing to be concerned about. She still looked upset, and told me that most of it was in the bathtub. I was beginning to get a little flustered with her because I didn't understand why this mattered, so I politely told her she would have to gather it up and then call housekeeping to come and clean the bathtub. She still looked a little freaked out, so I went to see Chad. There he sat, looking proud, because he had just pulled out all the hair along the middle of his head, thus achieving the reverse Mohawk. Sometimes he would pull it out in sections. I learned to warn the students about Chad's antics, but I could never bring myself to ask him not to do it.

Chad also loved to tease me mercilessly about my dating situation. I had been dating the same man for about three years when I met Chad. He was very probing in his questions, and didn't like my answer about why Lee and I were not engaged after three years. He loved to say "Well he's not going to buy the cow if he's getting free milk." Every time he would get admitted to the hospital he would ask "Has he bought the cow yet?" Or "Still giving free milk?" Chad came to my wedding in May 2003 with a pregnant Rachel, and one of my fondest memories and pictures in my wedding album is him holding the stick for the conga line.

After Chad stopped coming to Piedmont for treatments, we would keep in touch by email. I loved getting baby pictures of Kiersten, who is a mini Chad. He looked so happy in his life with Rachel and the baby. I was so grateful to God for giving Rachel such a beautiful baby to carry part of Chad with her every day.

When I got Rachel's email that Chad had passed away in spring 2005, I just felt deflated. Chad had lived longer than most of my patients with AML, mostly because of his amazing spirit and attitude and sheer will to live. I still have Chad's website saved to my favorites list, and the main page sums it all up: there's a picture of a man shooting a bird at

Death, and Chad has written underneath it "*My way of looking at leukemia!*"

In my job you care for so many people. One would think you couldn't keep track of them all. That's just not true. Cancer is a terrible disease, but these patients are the most motivated, determined people I have ever met. People ask me all the time, "How do you work in that environment?" Easy. I have the best job in the world. I get to take care of amazing people who make me go home every day and thank God for my health and everything around me. I am so grateful I was lucky enough to know Chad and be a part of his determined battle. To know him was to love him, and now I remember him and laugh when I think of him. I have my conga picture; I'll cherish it always.

Elizabeth

I met Chad at Northside Hospital where I coordinated his bone marrow transplant from an unrelated donor. (Of note, these "unrelated donors" are anonymous volunteer donors found in the National Marrow Donor Program, and could live anywhere in the world.) He was relentless in finding out who his donor was.

"What's his name?"
"Chad, I can't tell you."
"Is it a she?"
"Uhm, Chad I don't know."
"Is he OR she BLOND? Am I going to be blond? 'Cause that would be great."
"Uhm, Chad, maybe."
"Do you know where IT lives?"
"Uhm, Chad, I do. But I still can't tell you."
"Can you please just give me a clue?"
"Uh, no."
"Is it the U.S.? Germany?"
"Actually, Chad, the Philippines. Yeah, that's right, you're about to look like me."

Did I mention he's relentless? And a fighter!!! He's forever an inspiration.

Riza

Angels are everywhere. Not only do they deliver messages but they also serve to protect, guide and inspire.

I know Chad is watching over everyone he loves, especially his little girl. He was loved by many people and he is in our hearts. He touched so many people with his sense of humor, his orneriness, his smile and his compassion but, most of all, his bravery to continue. He never gave up. He will never be forgotten.

"Aunt Lisa"

Memories of Chad

I don't recall the first time that I met Chad. I worked closely with his mother Debbie and always knew she had two sons. We often saw each other and did things together when we lived in Hays, Kansas.

My sister and I were able to attend Chad's 21st birthday party, on Wednesday, February 25, 1998. The bar we had the celebration in was owned and ran by Chad's cousin. Many of the local family and friends were in attendance. He received a cake with a guitar on it and he got to imbibe in his first "legal" drink. Chad always had a passion for music, guitars, family, friends, fun and living life to the fullest.

One evening, Debbie and I went to a different local bar. Chad lived in Hays at that time and was there also. He asked me if I wanted to dance. I figured, "Sure why not?" I felt honored that he would want to dance with his mom's friend, but on the same token I felt like an aunt to him. Little did I know that they would start music for Mosh Pit dancing for the younger crowd. Lucky for me that Chad was so considerate and a gentleman, he would put his arms out and protect me from getting hit or slammed into. I can't say that I have done any Mosh Pit dancing since. It is a fond memory of Chad's fun side, attitude and gentlemanly manners.

As a vo-tech graduation gift to Chad, Debbie scheduled a trip to Cancun for him. It was a ritual for Debbie and his aunt Tina to go and enjoy the sun and beach there periodically. The trip would allow for six people. Shawn, his younger brother, decided to decline. He was not fond of the idea of traveling outside the United States; plus he didn't want to fly. There were only five of us that went: Chad, his vo-tech buddy, his aunt Tina, his mom and me. On May 29th we took off on our grand adventure. We drove two vehicles; both were small and would not hold all of us and the luggage. Debbie wanted to drive with the top down on her convertible, so we girls got a bit of a tan on the trip to Dallas. The boys wanted their space and not to be with us "old women." I enjoyed watching their many antics, including hanging their feet out the sides of the windows of the car while driving down interstate. We picked up Tina in Salina and we drove to Oklahoma and spent the night with a close friend of Debbie's, then on to Dallas. In Dallas we ate at a restaurant with a jungle theme and stayed at the motel and swam in the pool. We also practiced snorkeling since it was one of the many activities we planned for the clear Caribbean waters. The pool bottom was not nice to my nose, as I bumped and scraped it. Our plane was to leave at 8 am Sunday, May 31, 1998. While waiting in the parking lot for the airport shuttle, the boys enjoyed some hacky-sack games. We checked in, went to the pool and ocean, played water volleyball, ate at the Hard Rock Café for supper the first evening, and then partied at Tequila Sunrise. After partying we did some beach combing for shells and coral. The second day consisted of breakfast at the hotel, shopping in downtown Cancun, swimming and more sun several times. We ate American food that we recognized at Burger King for lunch. Senior Frogs was our venue for supper, *many great memories from that. We were in a crowd of many high school and college kids; we observed many of them splashing down the water slide into the ocean. Chad and his friend were very happily enjoying the long tall plastic tube glasses of refreshing drinks. Our hostess/waiter also had a fun buzzer game that we enjoyed trying to figure out. Tuesday was more of the beach, shopping, sun, etc. We went to Pirate Night, a Pirate Ship Party Cruise Adventure for the evening until after midnight. We all had our faces painted like pirates before we were allowed to board the ship. Chad was picked out of the crowd, participated in a limbo contest and danced the hula wearing a grass skirt. He was so much fun. Wednesday was a fun time going to Xel-Ha, we enjoyed the tubing down the river and snorkeling. We even got a picture of what looks like a barracuda, just inches away from our face and camera. More beach combing, talking to the parrot, watching spray paint art at night and dancing at the various clubs. Our many adventures in Cancun hold fond memories of Chad for me. After landing in Dallas and driving part way home we ran into a huge gully-washer rainstorm in Gainesville, Texas. It almost swept away the car the boys were driving. Again we stayed in Oklahoma and drove back home the next day.*

On September 27, 1998, I had four tickets to go to one of my favorite artist's hard rock concert in Kansas City. I had two tickets for me and two for my sister. As it turned out her friend canceled at the last minute. I was beside myself to try to find someone that could go with us; I didn't want to waste the ticket. Debbie suggested I try to get a hold of Chad, since he was living in KC at the time. We tried the day before the concert and the whole day of the concert while we traveled there. The concert started at 8 p.m. and we finally contacted him at 5:30 p.m. Chad brought a friend to the concert also. We had an awesome time listening to the warm up band which played heavy metal rock music and of course my favorite artist always puts on a good show. We sat around in the parking lot as the crowd died down and enjoyed the conversation amongst ourselves and passersby. Chad didn't know a stranger; everyone was his friend or a new acquaintance.

Looking back, I wonder if God was talking to me, when I had to decline taking a trip to Georgia with Debbie, in May 2001. She was going to visit Chad and Rachael in Georgia. I had many other obligations and was not able to take more time off that month. He was not feeling his best during her visit and she made a doctor's appointment for him while she was there. After many trips to the various doctors, and upon Debbie returning and a short time elapsing, we found out the fate of our sweet Chad. This is when the leukemia presented itself to us.

I had full intentions on attending Chad and Rachael's wedding in Arnold, Missouri, on June 1, 2002. He is like a brother, a nephew and a son to me. Then within a week I got another invitation to my own brother's wedding on the exact same day over 1100 miles away. Logistically, I could not make it to both. I was very excited that they were to become man and wife; it is a true bond that means so much in a person's life.

My last trip to Georgia before Chad died was January 16–19, 2005. I stayed with Chad, Rachael, Kiersten and Debbie in their Atlanta home. It was so good to see and talk to Chad during this visit, Chad was in pain but generally his normal self. Even though Debbie had always kept me up to date to his condition, he tried to explain to me the medical conditions of his eyes and body. He had GVH in his eyes at the time. I felt very privileged to be able to attend and witness a medical procedure that Chad had done during my stay in Atlanta. I was allowed by Chad to be in the room with him and watch the bone marrow biopsy/extraction for the tests they needed at that time. They took out more than required on the bone and bone marrow for the tests. He really was feeling the effects of the biopsy for many days after the procedure. Sadly, Chad only survived for two more months. It was the last time I saw him alive. I cherish the time I did get to spend with him and his family, witnessing his interactions with his wife, his child, his mother and me as a *friend. I have a very fond mental picture in my head of him resting with a kitty pillow and plush blanket I made for him and his family. We had many good times and laughs during that stay.*

I am sure when Chad and his guitars rolled into Heaven; he performed a very nice concert or jam session for God and the angels.

He was a truly unique individual and was very loved by many people. He is deeply missed.

Lisa (from Missouri)

I guess I should start in the beginning. Chad's mom and I have been best friends from the first day that we met. We were in our late teens, both married early. Both had our first children within a year or two of each other. She was "Aunt Debbie" to my girls and I was "Aunt Elaine" to her boys. We treated each other's kids like our own...complete to getting after them like we would our own. That being said, on with the story.

Chad. What a kid! From the day he was born with his blue eyes and blond hair, you could tell that he was going to be quite a kid. A true boy in every sense. You could just see the orneriness in those big blue eyes! They just twinkled. His grin filled the world with laughter and light.

And stubborn...oh my Lord. I remember when Debbie and I took all the kids to the Oklahoma State Fair. The boys were about 4 and 9 years old I think. We got there pretty early in the evening; maybe late, late afternoon was more like it. Anyway we had Chad and Shawn and my two girls. We had walked until we were pooped. We had seen everything there was to see and we "mommies" were ready to take our youngins home. However, the boys were not ready to go home and boy did we hear about it. They complained all the way back to the car that they wanted to go down the midway and ride the rides. Of course we went through why they couldn't do that. We even promised them

McDonald's, but they weren't going to hear of it. Chad was the most verbal about it as he was older than Shawn. He was very persistent that we should go back and go down the midway. We listened to him all the way back to the car and it was a looooong walk back to the car. We finally got there and Debbie got the boys strapped into their seatbelts, all the while trying to get them to hush up. It wasn't working. I got the stroller loaded and my little one in her car seat and my oldest in her seatbelt. I finally had had enough. I explained to them once more about "why" and told them to shut up or else I'd paddle their little hinnies for them. It's funny how kids will listen to someone other than their parent. Maybe it's the fear of God when somebody else gets after them. Either way, it worked and it was quiet from there on.

Incidents like this demonstrate the stubbornness and persistence that Chad had. He didn't give up easily, especially if he thought it was something worth fighting for. He loved moto-cross as a young boy and it didn't make any difference how banged up he got; he just went back for more.

He grew to be a wonderful young man. He loved his wife and child. He loved his brother and his mother and everyone around him. He was a good father and a good husband, a good brother and a good son.

Chad got a lot of his fortitude and persistence from his mother. Debbie is about the toughest ol' girl I know. I'm not sure I could have handled all she has gone through with Chad. He also got his faith in God from his mother. She taught him well. I'm a firm believer that Chad's stubbornness, persistence, fortitude and his faith in God more than anything are what helped him to beat his leukemia as long as he was able to. He just didn't give up easily.

It was a joy to know Chad and to love him and I miss him greatly. But in the end, he sits watching over us. His smile reflects in the sun, his warmth in the sand on the beach and his voice on the ocean waves.

Elaine

My Dear Son,

When I asked if anyone wanted to write a letter for the book to honor you, everyone stated that they could write a book themselves on just how wonderful and courageous you are. Many are feeling such a void since you departed that they cannot put into words on paper what they feel in their heart, mostly, your brother. You know, they were absolutely right. I have just finished writing this book and it is the second hardest thing I have ever had to do, second to losing you. There is still so much to say that is in my heart.

Before you were born I sat in church on Sundays with tears rolling down my cheeks in silence. So often I prayed for God to send me a child. I was once told by my very dear friend in Oklahoma, when you were just a few years old, that it was not your time to come to earth but you saw me crying. You asked God if you could come to earth early and be my child. You were always sensitive to others' feelings. I thank God and you for that and I thank my friend for telling me this back then. Thank you for picking me to be blessed as your mother. Perhaps that is why I had to let you go back home to God so early.

As you grew there were no terrible twos or horrible threes that other mothers kept telling me about, honestly. We had such a strong bonding between the two of us and our world was great. Later a brother was added to our family and our world became even more wonderful. Shawn was just what we needed to make things complete. The two of you had so much fun together. Please see over him as he still deals with so much anger and pain in missing you. I know you are as proud as I am of him at the person he has become.

As I watched you grow you held such responsibility and honor for your age. Yes, there were those things you did that you thought I did not know about. Later you found out Mom knew all along. I may not have approved of some of your life's lessons and experiences but I never, for one second, ever stopped loving you. I knew God was helping me in raising you to be a great young man. You knew of God and you knew of unconditional love and displayed them both in your life.

It was a joy to see your face as we traveled to new places. It gave me some of my most precious memories. You did the limbo in a grass skirt and snorkeled in Mexico, learned to scuba dive in Wisconsin, you learned to water ski in the Chocolate Bayou in Texas, saw Graceland in Tennessee, the Corn Castle and Yellowstone National Park, went to Disneyland in California, you ice fished and camped out in Alaska, and visited so many other places. There were more places you wanted to visit and now you can see them all from Heaven whenever you want.

You blessed me with a daughter when you married Rachael. You and she gave me one of the most precious gifts of all time, a granddaughter. Kiersten is your image in a mirror. She not only looks like you did at her age but she also has so many of your wonderful traits. Rachael is doing a wonderful job in raising her. I will do my best to help raise her to be as fine a person as you were. To have a part of you still here with us has saved me from totally falling apart. I will help her to know who you are.

A part of me died the same time you did. It will never return until I see you again and hold you in my arms. Forgive me if there was something I should have done or said to help you survive or ease your battle and did not.

In my selfishness, I was angry for you leaving but I eventually realized your peace after you passed on to live in Heaven with God. I miss you terribly and my heart still aches sometimes as it did the day you left. Just know that you are in my thoughts and heart each and every day and that I will someday be there to give you one of my hugs, scratch your head and rub your feet.

My love for you continues forever,
Mom

Chapter 34
March 24, 2006

Time to Go

The time had come for me to go
Yet I will be with you, this I know
Only in body did I leave
Because my life with yours I did weave
There is a part of me inside each of you
Know that I feel you inside me too
So take care of me while my body is gone
Share of the love with each day's new dawn
Know that with my love I leave you so many things
From comfort to strength I hope to you it brings
When you are down and need a gentle hand
Know that I am touching you from Heaven, where I am
If you feel as lonesome as you can be
Know that my heart is with you wherever you be
If you miss the times I could have been there
Know that every second of my life for you I do care
If you miss those smiles and laughter in the morn
Know that they are in the sunrise as each day is born
If you miss the hugs we shared at night
Know that I am closing my eyes and holding you tight
When you hurt or are sad and blue
On a breeze, a kiss I will send to you
Just remember that I have not died
I have only moved to the other side
A place I have prepared with me for you
It is a wonderful place to start anew

It has been one year since Chad passed away to live in Heaven with our Lord. I still carry the pain but have been learning better to deal with it. Our lives will never be the same. He will never be forgotten in all our hearts and minds. He taught us all some very valuable lessons about life. At times, as I remember the past, I think my heart will explode as it still hurts so badly.

One of Chad's favorite things to tell us all was, "Don't sweat the small stuff. It really doesn't matter."

As time continues to pass I have also found strength to rebuild my faith. Through reading the Bible and speaking with family and friends that are believers, I have found new comfort. I know in my heart that there is a Heaven where Chad lives and it is a wonderful place. I know this because Jesus would not have gone through all He went through and suffered on the cross as He did for us if there were not a Heaven. Someone once said to imagine the joys of Heaven and all its wondrous glory and arriving to run to Jesus and being held in His arms.

I strive and struggle with each day here on earth, as we all do. My faith will stand strong with the help of the Lord and one day I will join Chad in Heaven. I cannot wait for the day that I look into his sea blue eyes once more, give him a hug, rub his feet and scratch his head for him.

My joy now in my heart comes from seeing Chad in the sea blue eyes of Kiersten. She looks and acts like her father did. Her personality is exciting and she is full of love and joy.

We will always keep Chad alive for her. We will share with her the wonderful memories of her father. It is to her this book is truly dedicated.

If you are walking in those shoes or are a family or friend to someone who is, be their strength for them. Look to God and do not give up even in the bitter end. Use this book as a reminder that you are not alone and I hope to see you in Heaven.

I never took off the butterfly bracelet. It was removed from me by unseen hands (the clasp came apart) and fell off my wrist without my awareness and its whereabouts are not known. Perhaps some day I will find another. Perhaps this was part of Chad's way of telling me to release him and move on with my life and let others do so also. As I strive to do this I will still hold Chad dearly in my heart and mind and never forget him or the lessons about life that he has taught us all. Unconditional love is what it is all about.

I would like to bring this book to an end with a poem to all its readers. It was written on the first anniversary of Chad's death. I was told by the people I sent it to that it must be included in this book.

One Last Hug

Stop what you are doing on this busy day
And give your child a hug for me today
The most precious gift you will ever receive
As timeless memories in your life they weave

Forgive them for the things they broke
And for hurtful words they might have spoke
Speak encouraging words for their dreams
For time slips by all too quickly it seems

Whisper "I love you" in their ear
As you hold that precious child so dear
Teach them to follow God's given way
To live throughout each and every day

It was one year ago today
Angels came and took my son away
What I would give for a hug, just one more
Will have to wait for me to reach Heaven's door

Printed in the United States
107441LV00003B/172-177/A